T0147631

Skin Sense!

Skin Sense!

*

A Dermatologist's Guide
to
Skin and Facial Care; Third Edition

Stephen M. Schleicher, MD

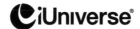

Skin Sense!
A Dermatologist's Guide to Skin and Facial Care; Third Edition

iUniverse books may be ordered through booksellers or by contacting:

iUniverse
1663 Liberty Drive
Bloomington, IN 47403
www.iuniverse.com
1-800-Authors (1-800-288-4677)

Because of the dynamic nature of the Internet, any web addresses or links contained in this book may have changed since publication and may no longer be valid. The views expressed in this work are solely those of the author and do not necessarily reflect the views of the publisher, and the publisher hereby disclaims any responsibility for them.

ISBN: 978-1-4401-7427-8 (sc)
ISBN: 978-1-4401-7426-1 (hc)
ISBN: 978-1-4401-7428-5 (e)

Print information available on the last page.

iUniverse rev. date: 11/20/2017

Contents

ABOUT THE AUTHOR

Dr. Schleicher brings over twenty years of experience in the field of dermatology. He graduated Phi Beta Kappa from Rutgers University, received his medical degree with academic honors from the Hahnemann Medical College and completed his dermatology residency at the Temple Skin and Cancer Hospital. The author of three books and over one hundred journal articles, Dr. Schleicher served for over a decade on the Editorial Board of Emergency Medicine magazine and on the Advisory Board of the Day Spa Association. He has travelled to both Europe and Brazil investigating skin care products for pharmaceutical and cosmetic industries. He has also served as a Principal Investigator for over three dozen phase III and phase IV clinical studies. A pioneer in the field of teledermatology, Dr. Schleicher was named a ComputerWorld Honors Laureate in 2011, this an international competition recognizing "men and women whose visionary applications of information technology promote positive social, economic and educational change." Also in 2011 Dr. Schleicher received the Innovators Award from the Pennsylvania Medical Society which featured his trailblazing work in the field of telemedicine. Dr. Schleicher founded the DermDOX Center for Teledermatology (dermdox. org) and the DermDox Centers for Dermatology (www.dermdoxcenters.com). He is an Associate Professor of Medicine at the Commonwealth Medical College, an Adjunct Assistant Professor of Dermatology at the University of Pennsylvania Medical College, and a Clinical Instructor of dermatology at the physician assistant divisions of Kings College and Arcadia, Marywood and Misericordia Universities.

INTRODUCTION

Introducing … skin! The incredibly durable outermost layer of the human body. Akin to the turtle's shell or an armadillo's plate, this essential overcoat forms a protective seal that insulates delicate structures from the environment and shields us from physical injury, temperature changes, solar radiation, harmful chemicals, and dangerous microorganisms. Yet skin functions not only to protect; it also serves to beautify. Skin is an inescapable source of our self-consciousness, attractiveness, and vanity. We often look at, touch, and caress our own skin and that of others. For those enmeshed in a superficial, glittering, image-conscious society, beauty does indeed become but skin deep. Skin mirrors and shapes our very emotions: it blushes, radiates, glistens, and sweats. Skin conveys and transmits supreme pleasure and agonizing pain. We are bound by our skin, physically and, in many ways, psychologically.

The stamina of this remarkable tissue is incredible. During much of our existence we unknowingly torment our skin. The body is washed daily with any number of chemicals and then coated with a slew of substances ranging from mass-produced cosmetics to synthetic antiperspirants. In the winter we rush from heated, humidity-depleted buildings into sub-zero temperatures. In the summer we gleefully roast under the suns heat and penetrating rays. We dive into chlorinated pools and frolic in salt-laden oceans.

Just how enduring is skin? If one were to take the unpainted sheet-metal frame of an automobile and expose it to the same environment that confronts our body, within weeks one would be left with a rusted, rotting piece of junk. Yet skin lasts a lifetime!

The key to skin's durability is its amazing regenerative power. Skin is composed of billions of living cells. As soon as one of these cells becomes injured or dies, a new one rushes to take its place. Such is the natural process of healing, and because of this biological phenomenon, any damage to our outer shell is usually temporary. Usually.

As we shall see, there are times when even our skin has had enough. Skin disease affects 1 in 4 Americans and the prevalence increases as our population ages. The number of patients with skin disease exceeds those with heart disease or diabetes.

NORMAL SKIN

Our skin, the cutaneous organ, is composed of three distinct layers: the epidermis, the dermis, and subcutaneous (or fat) tissue. The following brief descriptions of each layer will greatly aid in the understanding of both healthy and diseased skin.

The epidermis constitutes the outermost layer and is the only part of the skin that is visible to us. From a cosmetic standpoint, the epidermis is naturally of paramount importance.

The epidermis is the thinnest of all layers and over much of our body it is only one-sixteenth of an inch thick, about as thick as this page. The epidermis is thickest on the palms and soles, where it may reach nearly one-eighth of an inch.

The epidermis is composed of both living and dead cells. New cells are produced in the lowest portion, the basal layer. These cells migrate upward to the surface to become the cornified layer. Here the cells form a resilient, waterproof material known as keratin. Dead surface cells are continuously shed as miniscule flakes (scales) and are immediately replaced by living cells from the layers below. Some twenty-eight days are required for a new cell produced in the basal layer to finally reach the outer cornified zone; in other words, complete replacement of the epidermis takes nearly one month.

The epidermis is devoid of blood vessels. This alone gives some indication of the thinness of this layer, for we all have experienced bleeding following a superficial nick or cut. Thus even the most trivial of wounds easily traverse the thin epidermis to enter the next layer, the dermis.

The dermis is some forty times thicker than the epidermis. Besides harboring blood vessels, it also contains nerves, sweat glands, and sebaceous oil glands. The dermis feeds the cells of the basal layer and consequently regulates the growth of the entire epidermis. Tautness of the skin is in large part due to components such as collagen and elastin fibers that reside in the dermis.

The dermis rests on a thick pad of fat called the subcutaneous layer. This layer, like the epidermis, varies in thickness depending on body location. It is practically nonexistent within the eyelid and, as you might guess, becomes thickest around the waist (too thick in some cases!). The subcutaneous tissue serves as a thermal insulator and shock absorber.

Unhealthy skin may result from a disease process that affects any or all of the three layers. For example, dry skin involves changes in the epidermis; acne is a disorder of sebaceous glands located in the dermis; and cellulite arises from alterations in the subcutaneous tissue.

Male and Female Skin

So, is male skin from Mars and female skin from Venus? Hopefully, we are all Earthlings, but differences in the sexes certainly carry over to our skin as well. Male skin is indeed thicker than female skin. Increased collagen and elastin fibers in men contribute to firmness and are a main reason why men tend to age with fewer deep-set wrinkles and fine lines than women. Another reason for aging disparity is the fact that male skin has a greater number of coarse hair follicles. Over time, exposure to solar radiation breaks down dermal collagen and contributes mightily to wrinkle formation, but facial hair (the male beard) acts as a physical screen to ultraviolet light.

Male skin has more active oil and sweat-gland activity than female skin; thus men have less need to moisturize. Bacteria living on the skin surface degrade sweat, leading to the characteristic musty aroma of the male armpit and the enhanced need for deodorants (at least when out in public!).

The placement of fat is to some degree sex-related and varies in males and females. The distribution in women gives rise to the more rounded contours associated with the feminine figure and in large part contributes to culturally defined "sexiness."

Black and White Skin

Pigment cells within the skin are called melanocytes, and the actual pigment is known as melanin. Melanin production varies among the various cultural groups, including Africans, Asians, and Caucasians. Interestingly, black skin does not contain more melanocytes, but it does tend to contain more melanin. The melanin granules are larger and darker.

Variations in human skin color have evolved over the ages. Black skin is the most resistant to ultraviolet light and is ideally suited to withstand chronic sun exposure. Indeed, unprotected white or pale skin is a sitting duck for skin cancer.

A redeeming feature of sunlight is that it induces production of vitamin D, which is extremely important for our health and well-being. Thus melanin serves as a double-edged sword. By blocking solar radiation, melanin protects against skin cancer, but it also inhibits vitamin D production. One can postulate that as humans migrated from sunnier climates to colder ones, skin lightening was a positive adaptation to a changing environment. The need for melanin to prevent skin cancer lessened with decreased sun exposure, and decreased amounts of melanin actually enhanced vitamin D production by skin cells.

NUTRITION AND THE SKIN

Three main food types are essential in the everyday maintenance of our body. These are carbohydrates, proteins, and fats, all of which contribute to healthy skin.

Despite occasional pitches to the contrary, a "superskin" diet has yet to be developed. Perhaps one day what we eat will indeed serve as a fountain of youth that thwarts the aging process. For now one would do best to follow the sound nutritional principles that medical doctors advocate for the majority of the population: a diet low in calories, high in fiber and whole grains, and moderate in saturated fats with reduced levels of salt and sugar.

The role of diet in causing or perpetuating our most common skin conditions is somewhat controversial. A diet rich in fat does not make the skin oilier, and drinking large amounts of fluid will not put moisture back into the skin. Does chocolate worsen breakouts? Possibly. Recent data suggests that eating refined carbohydrates and sugar leads to a surge in an insulin-like growth factor that triggers an excess of male hormones. Male hormones signal skin cells to excrete large amounts of sebum (oil). Increased sebum production is a contributing factor to pimple formation. An even stronger association has been made with milk; cow hormones present in milk have been linked to the development of acne.

On occasion one may become allergic to a particular food or food additive, resulting in hives. Common offenders include strawberries and shellfish. And one uncommon skin disease, called dermatitis herpetiformis, is actually linked to sensitivity to gluten, which is found in many foods, including bread and beer.

Marked fluctuations in weight may also affect the skin. Gaining pounds augments the amount of body fat, which in turn predisposes a person to stretch marks and cellulite. Rapid weight loss (from crash dieting, for example) may result in decreased skin turgor and may actually aggravate the cosmetic disfigurement that accompanies cellulite.

Vitamins and minerals are substances found in our food (and medicine cabinets) that are required in minute quantities for proper maintenance of the body. Botanicals are compounds that contain extracts or active ingredients derived from plants. Nutraceuticals are products that have been isolated or purified from food and are used for medicinal purposes. In regard to skin care, vitamins, minerals, botanicals, and nutraceuticals are utilized either internally (taken by mouth) or topically (placed on the skin). There is still much to be learned about the action and effects of these substances, and this most certainly contributes to the multitude of inflated claims associated with their use.

From the standpoint of our skin, one should note that substances such as minerals and vitamins, so essential to the human body in trace amounts, may or may not have beneficial effects when chemically modified or used in higher concentrations. One should note as well that the labeling of an herbal or botanical product as "natural" or "organic" means nothing in regard to efficacy. And the fact that something comes from a plant does *not* make it safe or effective—take tobacco and poison ivy, for example.

Vitamin A

Vitamin A is a fat-soluble vitamin that plays a very important role in maintaining healthy skin. The substance is found in certain food items such as eggs, whole milk, and liver, and it is added to fat-free milk and many cereals. Retinol is an active form of the vitamin, and beta-carotene (found in green leafy vegetables) is a vitamin A precursor.

In the United States, vitamin A deficiency is a rare occurrence. An excess of this vitamin is usually the result of dietary supplement overindulgence. Because vitamin A is fat-soluble, it can be stored in the body and can accumulate in harmful levels. Too much vitamin A can damage the liver and may contribute to osteoporosis. Signs of acute toxicity included nausea, vomiting, headache, and visual disturbances. Pregnant women should avoid vitamin A supplementation since the substance is a known teratogen (inducer of birth defects).

Topical and oral vitamin A-based compounds are used to treat acne and psoriasis. Two FDA-approved derivatives, Renova and Avage, may diminish fine lines and wrinkles. The vitamin A compounds retinol and retinyl palmitate are found in over-the-counter products, and these too may improve the appearance of aging skin. Clinical trials comparing the efficacy of the prescription and nonprescription topical formulations of this vitamin are still lacking.

Biotin

Biotin is a water-soluble B vitamin necessary for metabolism and growth. The compound is found in many foods including liver, soy products, carrots, and cereals. Deficiency is rare and curiously may be induced by a diet rich in raw eggs, as a substance in egg whites prevents intestinal absorption of the vitamin. The first signs of biotin deficiency involve the hair and nails, which lose luster and become brittle. Thus, intuitively, some believe that excess biotin (in pill form) will in fact strengthen these integuments. Biotin given to horses appears to enhance hoof quality, and anecdotal evidence in humans suggests that it may be of benefit to our hair and nails.

Vitamin C

Vitamin C (ascorbic acid) is a water-soluble vitamin that plays a key role in the formation of collagen, a substance necessary for healthy bones, cartilage, muscle, and blood vessels. This vitamin is acquired mostly by eating fruits and vegetables, and healthy individuals who eat balanced diets rarely need supplementation. Vitamin C deficiency (extraordinarily rare in the United States) leads to a condition called scurvy, which is characterized by joint pains, muscle weakness, gum bleeding, and skin lesions. Except for gastric irritation, oral intake of large amounts of the vitamin does not appear to have serious consequences, nor does it appear to have much benefit despite at one time being touted as a cure for the common cold and a preventative of cancer.

Of late, vitamin C has been incorporated into a variety of over-the-counter preparations touting anti-aging and anti-inflammatory properties. Vitamin C is a powerful antioxidant that may, when used topically, stimulate collagen production and offer some level of protection against the damaging effects of sunlight. The problem is that vitamin C in topical formulations is highly unstable and rapidly breaks down when exposed to the environment (which is why most products are packaged in dark containers). More documentation of the stability, skin-penetrating abilities, and efficacy of currently marketed products is needed before they can be recommended from a therapeutic standpoint; but many vitamin C products are well tolerated and are formulated within elegant, moisturizing bases.

Vitamin D

Vitamin D is a very hot topic, as a significant percentage of elderly Americans are deficient in this vitamin, and low levels are linked to osteoporosis and, less convincingly, to heart disease and cancer. The Institute of Medicine recommends that adults should receive 600 IU of vitamin D daily and those above age 70 should receive 800 IU. Vitamin D is found in fortified milk, fatty fish such as salmon, and in dietary supplements. It is also produced in the skin upon exposure to sun and ultraviolet light; hence it is called the "sunshine vitamin." Lighter skin produces more vitamin D than darker skin. Just five minutes outdoors three times weekly allows many individuals to produce the necessary amount of this vitamin. However, dietary supplementation is highly recommended for those who cannot tolerate the sun, give a family or personal history of skin cancer, lack access to sunlight, are elderly, or have darker complexions.

Vitamin E

Vitamin E is a fat-soluble vitamin found naturally in vegetable oils, nuts, and green leafy vegetables. Deficiency of this vitamin is quite rare, and the merits of supplementation are contested. Indeed, vitamin E is a marvelous example of the hype associated with antioxidants and the aging process. Thirty years ago this vitamin was trumpeted as a retardant of cellular demise helping to gobble up damaging free radicals, the harmful byproducts of metabolism and sun exposure. Megadoses were in vogue. No longer. As far back as 1994 the American Heart Association warned that high doses of vitamin E could actually increase the risk of death, and a study published in 2009 found no evidence that it prevented cancer. Further, a 2014 study demonstrated that men taking high-dose Vitamin E supplements doubled their risk of prostate cancer.

Vitamin E has been used for decades as an ingredient in certain over-the-counter treatments for dry skin, and more recently, for its postulated anti-aging properties. Topical vitamin E (in the form of either alpha tocopherol or tocopherol acetate) has antioxidant properties, which in animal models protect epidermal cells from environmental damage such as that caused by sunlight.

To date, human studies are inconclusive, perhaps in part because this vitamin, like vitamin C, has difficulty penetrating the skin.

Vitamin K

Vitamin K is a fat-soluble vitamin which helps activate the clotting mechanism of our blood. This vitamin is found in cabbage, green leafy vegetables such as spinach, and soybeans. Deficiency of this vitamin may be induced by diseases that interfere with intestinal absorption, but is quite rare.

Several topical formulations contain vitamin K and claim to reduce the severity of bruising, diminish the appearance of tiny leg veins, and even improve dark circles under the eyes. Very little scientific data substantiates any of these claims, although one small study using topical vitamin K reported diminished bruising following laser treatment for facial blood vessels.

Zinc

Zinc is an essential mineral that has diverse physiological functions and plays a critical role with enzymes and proteins needed to maintain healthy skin. It is found in abundance in beef, pork, lamb, and peanuts. Dietary deficiency of zinc is very unusual in the United States. Certain rare genetic disorders are characterized by the inability to absorb zinc, resulting in inflamed skin and rashes. Topical zinc has anti-inflammatory and antibacterial properties and is incorporated into shampoos (for example, DHS Zinc and Head & Shoulders Extra Strength) to control dandruff. Oral zinc supplementation has been reported to improve acne, although evidence of a beneficial effect is far from convincing. In doses greater than 40 mg per day zinc can be toxic and supplementation has been linked to an increased risk of advanced prostate cancer as well as to reduced levels of HDL ("good") cholesterol.

Nicotinamide

Nicotinamide (or niacinamide) is a derivative of niacin, a component of the B vitamin complex. These compounds enable our cells to produce energy and also help repair damage to DNA induced by sun exposure. A deficiency of this vitamin is quite rare but leads to the condition known as pellagra, which is characterized by dementia and a skin rash. B vitamins are found in a variety of plant and animal food sources.

Application of nicotinamide to the skin may help prevent moisture loss and sun damage. Some data indicates that topical niacinamide has anti-inflammatory properties and may help to improve acne and rosacea.

Coenzyme Q$_{10}$

A skin care ingredient currently in vogue is coenzyme Q$_{10}$. Also called ubiquinone-10, this cellular antioxidant is located in all tissues of the body, including skin. The vitamin-like substance is found in organ meats such as heart, liver, and kidney, as well as in soybean oil and certain fish. Oral supplementation has been used as an adjunct to cancer therapy and in the management of Parkinson's disease and congestive heart failure.

Coenzyme Q$_{10}$ is now found in a variety of lotions and creams and is claimed to have anti-aging effects. The skin levels of this compound do appear to decrease naturally with age, and a small study demonstrated a beneficial effect on wrinkles about the eye.

Alpha Lipoic Acid

Alpha lipoic acid (ALA) is a potent antioxidant that helps to deactivate free radicals. It also has anti-inflammatory activity. ALA is found in only trace amounts in food. Oral supplementation has been used as treatment for diabetic neuropathy and Alzheimer's disease.

Topical preparations contain ALA in concentrations ranging from 1 percent to 5 percent. ALA is readily absorbed through the skin and apparently can enter the dermis and subcutaneous layers. A very small study showed encouraging results when used on sun-damaged skin.

Lycopene

Lycopene is an antioxidant found in high concentration in red tomatoes (including juice, sauce, paste, and ketchup). The substance appears to concentrate in certain organs including the prostate gland, colon, and skin. High intake of food substances containing lycopene is associated with a decreased risk of gastrointestinal and prostate cancer. Lycopene and related compounds (called carotenoids) may help protect the skin from ultraviolet light damage, and several commercially available creams incorporate this compound in conjunction with other vitamins. Claims that such products will boost collagen production or reduce wrinkles and crow's feet have not been substantiated.

Peptides

Peptides are compounds containing amino acids, which serve as the building blocks of proteins such as collagen. A few appear to aid in the healing of ulcers and wounds and are thought to do so by stimulating collagen production. Results of small industry-sponsored studies using a variety of peptides (some containing copper) demonstrate improvement of wrinkles and photoaging, and several facial lotions and eye creams containing peptides are on the market.

Growth Factors

Growth factors are a group of proteins that play a role in wound healing and tissue regeneration. Growth factors incorporated into skin creams and serums may come from a variety of sources including cell cultures, placental cells, and plants. Kinetin is a plant-derived growth factor that has antioxidant properties and retards the aging of certain cells. Kinetin lotions are in general non-irritating. Preliminary studies indicate that, like retinoids, growth factors may improve wrinkles and dark spots. However, skin cells do contain retinoid receptors, but not kinetin receptors, leaving the efficacy of this product in doubt.

Tea Extracts

Green tea, black tea, and oolong tea contain substances called polyphenols, which have significant antioxidant and anti-inflammatory activity. In animals and humans, application of a green-tea ointment appears to lessen the incidence of ultraviolet-induced skin cancers, and tea-derived polyphenols are now found in a number of skin care formulations. Anti-wrinkle and skin-smoothing claims have also been made. Determining the true benefit of topically applied tea extracts awaits the outcome of larger clinical studies.

Lecithin/Phosphatidylcholine

Lecithin and its purified derivative, phosphatidylcholine, are components of cell membranes. Choline, the major constituent of phosphatidylcholine, is found naturally in soybeans, oatmeal, liver, cabbage, and cauliflower. Several skin care formulations contain lecithin, used primarily for its moisturizing properties. A liquid form of phosphatidylcholine is often used in a procedure called mesotherapy, which attempts to melt away fat cells using injections into subcutaneous tissue. This drug is not approved for use in the United States, and the safety and efficacy of this procedure has not been documented.

Soy Proteins

Soybeans contain ingredients called flavonoids that are structurally related to the female hormone estrogen. Women with high dietary intake appear to have lessened risks of breast cancer and cardiovascular disease. Studies in mice demonstrate that topically applied soy protein protects against ultraviolet light and significantly decreases the occurrence of skin cancer. Soy proteins also show promise as skin-lightening and collagen-stimulating agents.

Aloe Vera

Aloe vera is one of the most widely used botanical products. The gel is found within the leaves of the aloe vera plant and consists of 99.5 percent water and a collection of polysaccharides. Aloe vera has been reported to increase blood flow, reduce inflammation, and promote healing, and it has been used to treat many skin diseases including eczema, psoriasis, and even genital herpes. Aloe is found in hundreds of over-the-counter preparations including moisturizers, soaps, sunscreens, and shampoos, but many contain concentrations so low that any therapeutic effect from this plant is quite dubious. Despite the widespread consumer use of aloe, there is a paucity of high-quality scientific research documenting its effectiveness other than as a run-of-the-mill moisturizer. In a 2008 study, aloe vera applied to burns did not speed regeneration of skin.

Pycnogenol

Pycnogenol is an extract made from the bark of French marine pine. The compound contains flavonoids and is claimed to prevent cardiovascular disease and decrease leg swelling when taken orally. Pycnogenol is an antioxidant and is incorporated into several skin creams, some of which claim sun-protection and anti-aging properties. But there is a dearth of scientific evidence supporting such claims.

CoffeeBerry extract

CoffeeBerry, derived from the crushed, processed fruit of the *Coffea arabica* plant, is another trendy antioxidant utilized in creams and purported to promote skin rejuvenation, environmental damage protection, and pigment reduction. Two small studies offer encouraging results, but more data is certainly needed to confirm that the claims are fact rather than just talk-show hype.

Grape seed extract

Grape seed extracts contain an ample supply of polyphenols. Although some are similar to those found in tea, others have distinct properties. Scientific data supports the antioxidant activities of these compounds, said to be more potent than vitamins C and E. When utilized within topical preparations, grape seed extracts are claimed to improve skin tone, prevent scars and stretch marks, hasten wound healing, and protect against sun damage. More clinical studies are needed to support such claims. Resveratrol is a potent antioxidant found in the skin of red grapes and red wine, which—in massive doses—may or may not prevent or reduce the ravages of cellular aging. Studies in mice are promising. However meaningful long term safety and efficacy data gleaned from human testing are several years away. Stay tuned.

Açai

Açai, the berry from the Brazilian palm, is another hot additive to skin care products. The compound contains potent antioxidants and is a rich source of the flavonoid anthocyanin, which is purported to protect the skin from free radicals, thereby retarding the aging process. Topical compounds are limited in concentration due to the propensity for skin staining, and to date, solid clinical studies documenting efficacy are lacking.

Turmeric

Turmeric is a spice commonly used in Asian and Indian foods. The biologically active component, curcumin, has documented anti-inflammatory properties. Topical application studies supports facilitation of wound healing and the prevention of skin cancer. Worldwide, especially in India, curcumin is often added to skin care preparations.

Coconut Oil

Coconut oil is another trending "super food" and one that contains a high level of short and medium chained saturated fats. The benefit of these substances on the cardiovascular system is highly contested and several organizations, including the American Heart Association, recommend consuming them in moderation. A study published in 2014 demonstrated that topically applied coconut oil improved eczema in pediatric patients with mild to moderate eczema.

DRY SKIN

Problems associated with dry skin rank among the most common complaints that a dermatologist deals with in daily practice. Over three hundred million dollars are spent each year on over-the-counter preparations in attempts to alleviate the annoying manifestations of moisture-depleted skin. Dry skin (also called xerosis) is the result of excessive water loss from the outermost layer of the epidermis, the stratum corneum. Signs of this condition become apparent when the skin has lost so much water that normal flexibility of this organ can no longer be maintained. Dry skin is characterized by roughness, chafing, cracking, and in more severe cases, by redness and inflammation.

The moisture content of the stratum corneum is in large part responsible for the normal appearance of the skin. The amount of moisture in this top layer is partially controlled by the relative humidity and temperature of the surrounding air. Rapid evaporation of water readily occurs in cold weather and at low humidity. For this reason, dry skin is most common during the winter months. Air conditioning and forced-air heating also promote skin dryness. As the skin loses moisture, tiny cracks appear on its surface, which is the initial stage of skin chapping.

Placing the skin in contact with water will not add moisture to the outer layer. In fact, this will have exactly the opposite effect. Too frequent bathing is a common contributing factor to the dry skin experienced by many of us. To help minimize the effects of environment and humidity on the skin, the body coats its surface with a protective mixture of sweat and oils produced by specialized glands in the dermis. Frequent washing, especially with harsh detergent soaps, removes this protection and permits the skin to dry out at an accelerated rate. Thus, showering or sitting in the tub more than once a day is discouraged for those afflicted with dry skin. These individuals should use lukewarm water, as hot water tends to be even more drying.

One might postulate that drinking ample fluids would replenish the moisture content of skin. This is certainly the advice recommended time and again by health and beauty magazine columnists. Too bad this is a myth.

Drinking five or six glasses of water a day is good for the kidneys but simply will not rehydrate the epidermis of a non-dehydrated human.

The best way to minimize and treat xerosis is through the use of moisturizers. Lubricating creams, lotions, and ointments work by forming a semi-occlusive film over the skin's surface thereby minimizing evaporative water loss. Emollients are agents that fill in spaces between skin cells, soothing rough skin. Ingredients that confer emollient properties include lanolin, butyl stearate, and petrolatum. Emollients are either water- or oil-based. In general, water-based moisturizers (such as Cetaphil-brand lotions) are easier to apply, and oil-based compounds (such as Eucerin-brand creams) are more occlusive and function longer. Some moisturizers contain ingredients that deposit substances called humectants on the skin surface, which helps the skin to absorb water. Examples of humectants include lactic acid, urea, and glycerin. Ammonium lactate contains alpha hydroxy acid and is available over-the counter (AmLactin, Lac-Hydrin Five) and, in higher strength, by prescription (Lac-Hydrin 12%).

The most inexpensive moisturizer is—believe it or not—Crisco. This vegetable oil will do a fine job of lubricating the skin at a very reasonable price. Most people, however, prefer not to keep a jar on the bathroom counter, hence cosmetic and drug companies today market scores of lubricants whose ultimate goals are skin moisturization and water-loss prevention. Also recommended are use of non-detergent, lubricating soaps and bath oils. People anticipating sun exposure should use moisturizers with sunscreen. Individuals with "normal" skin can use water-based products; those with dry skin do best with oil-based versions. (In general, the drier the skin, the thicker the required moisturizer.) People with sensitive skin should avoid fragranced formulations.

Relatively new to the market are moisturizers that help repair damaged skin barriers. Depletion of fatty acids (lipids) within the skin can result secondary to chemical and environmental assault and can also accompany the aging process. Compounds such as ceramides, stearic acid, and palmitic acid are substances that mimic those barriers found within the stratum corneum. Two nonprescription barrier repair compounds are Cerave and Restoraderm; prescription barrier repair agents include EpiCeram and Neosalus.

In sum, if you are plagued with dry skin, there are measures you can take to minimize this annoying problem. Avoid frequent washing and the use of harsh soaps, substituting instead lubricating cleansers especially formulated for sensitive skin. Bath oil should be added to each bath. After leaving the bath or shower, apply a moisturizing cream, lotion, or ointment, while the skin is still damp, to trap the film of water that coats the skin's surface. Moisturize frequently and in cold weather modify the environment by using a humidifier. Adhering to these simple procedures will go a long way toward improving skin that is rough, scaly, and flaky.

THE ACNE PROBLEM

Do zits give you fits? Chances are, yes. Acne is the most common skin problem affecting three out of every four teenagers to some degree. And an imperfect complexion is not limited to this age group; many in their twenties and thirties also suffer with this condition. The problem is an expensive one, with millions of dollars spent each year on over-the-counter preparations as well as prescription drugs. For many, acne consists of nothing more than an occasional pimple or blemish on the face, back, or chest. A few are less fortunate and develop extensive, persistent eruptions resulting in permanent pits and scars. The psychological effects may be devastating, and acne has been linked to depression and suicidal thoughts.

Acne is dependent on the presence of sebaceous (oil) glands found within the dermis of the skin. These specialized structures are most numerous on the face but are also present on the back, chest, and upper arms. At puberty the glands undergo rapid enlargement because of hormonal stimulation. As the glands grow in size they become more active, manufacturing a mixture of oils that in excessive amounts gives rise to the so-called oily complexion. The gland openings (pores) may become clogged, causing the oil, or sebum, to back up and stagnate. Bacteria growing in the sebum break down this substance into a number of irritating compounds that lead to the formation of blackheads, whiteheads, and those unsightly mountains and craters affectionately called zits.

There are several different types of acne lesions. These include comedones (whiteheads and blackheads), papules, pustules, cysts, and scars. Comedones are of two varieties: open and closed. A closed comedone, called a whitehead, arises when a pore becomes clogged with oil and the sebum creates a tiny white covering over the entrance. When the opening remains unobstructed, the oil is oxidized by the air and turns black. This open type of comedone is called a blackhead.

A papule is a solid, elevated lesion of the skin. Papules range in hue from flesh-colored to bright red. Red papules are those pimples still undergoing inflammation.

A pustule is a pimple filled with fluid, or pus. This substance is composed of dead cells and bacteria. When a pustule becomes larger and deeper, it is then termed a cyst. Tender, inflamed red pustules and cysts may result in scars, which is why these two types represent the most severe forms of acne.

What then is the cause of acne? Why is it that some people escape this condition entirely, while others are plagued with blemishes, zits, and blackheads year after year?

Acne appears to be the result of a number of factors; there is no single cause. Certainly a major factor is heredity. If one of your parents had acne, you run an increased risk of acquiring this condition.

Another contributing factor to the development of acne is the activity of certain hormones within the body. For many, acne first becomes a problem at puberty. During this period, testosterone, the male sex hormone, is formed not only by the male sex organs, but also in small quantities by the ovaries in young women. Testosterone causes marked growth of the sebaceous glands and, in susceptible persons, may trigger or worsen acne.

Some females develop one or two pimples each month shortly before their menstrual periods. Others may flare when placed on certain birth control pills. In both cases, the resultant acne is due to changes in the body's hormone levels. Polycystic ovary syndrome is characterized by irregular periods, excess facial hair, and scalp hair thinning. Abnormal hormone levels in women so afflicted results in persistent acne.

An increasing number of American women are developing acne not at puberty or in adolescence but during their twenties and thirties. Some attribute this phenomenon in part to the prolonged use of cosmetics. Moisturizers, creams, and cover-ups may lead to pore plugging and induction of comedones and papules. Others believe that the stresses of modern life subtly alter hormone levels which in turn triggers breakouts.

Certainly a major factor that contributes to acne at any age and in either sex is the bacteria that live within the sebaceous glands breaking down the skin's natural oils into irritating by-products. These bacteria and the substances they produce play a key role in the inflammatory lesions of acne.

Certain factors once thought to play a significant role in the cause and perpetuation of acne are now considered quite unimportant. No evidence exists that lack of regular washing leads to a worsening of acne. By the same token, acne does not appear to be improved by incessant cleansing. Washing two or three times daily is all that is usually needed to remove excess oil and germs on the skin's surface.

Lingering controversy surrounding acne involves the role of diet. A diet high in fats and oils does not make the skin oilier; greasy skin is not caused by greasy foods. A study conducted years ago was unable to demonstrate that feeding individuals with acne huge quantities of chocolate led to increased pimple formation. However, more recently, a link has been postulated between breakouts and high-glycemic-load diets that are rich in processed carbohydrates. Acne severity decreased in volunteers maintained on low-carbohydrate diets, but these diets also promoted weight loss, which alone may have triggered changes in body hormones that diminished the number of breakouts.

Speaking of hormones, yes, the role of milk in acne causation is also controversial. Again, a recent study found a positive association between milk intake and acne. Since the majority of milk comes from pregnant cows, a tenable hypothesis holds that hormones in milk have a stimulatory effect on the oil glands of those that drink it.

For most, acne merely represents a temporary embarrassment, while for some the condition constitutes a disfiguring disease. Regardless of the extent of involvement, virtually all cases will significantly improve with proper therapy.

Certain general principles are best followed when dealing with acne. As mentioned, it is advisable to wash the affected areas twice daily to remove excess sebum and bacteria from the skin's surface. Acne cleansers and soaps often contain surfactants that facilitate oil removal. Cleansers containing benzoyl peroxide and salicylic acid are very effective. Defatting solutions known as astringents may aid in the temporary removal of surface film. Abrasive cleansers contain fine granules that are rubbed against the skin to produce a mild "sandpaper" effect. Such preparations will help reduce excess oil but can cause increased peeling and may prove too harsh for some persons; dermatologists discourage their use in the inflammatory types of acne. Nonirritating, noncomedogenic soaps are recommended for those with sensitive skin.

Persons with acne must strenuously avoid picking, scratching, squeezing, or otherwise manipulating their pimple-plagued skin. Unless properly instructed, leave all mechanical manipulations to a skin care specialist. The temptation is certainly great to force out pus-bumps and to pop zits. But such facial trauma, besides coating the bathroom mirror, may transform an ordinary pimple into a permanent scar.

Sunlight often plays a beneficial role in acne treatment. Many people experience a considerable improvement in their complexion during the summer months. Of course, one must weigh this benefit against any harmful, long-term effects of ultraviolet radiation. Further, some acne therapies do not mix with sunlight.

Persons with acne usually try over-the-counter acne preparations as first-line treatment. Active ingredients may include sulfur, resorcinol, benzoyl peroxide, salicylic acid, or alcohol. All promote drying and peeling and help limit bacterial growth.

Those who do not respond to the above measures should consider medical consultation. Dermatologists possess considerable knowledge concerning the nature and course of acne and have at their disposal a number of powerful therapeutic modalities to improve one's appearance and—of equal importance—to prevent scars. Indeed, a good percentage of persons with acne require medical specialist treatment to prevent physical or psychological scarring.

Benzoyl Peroxide

One of the mainstays of acne therapy is application of benzoyl peroxide. Preparations containing this substance promote facial drying and are antibacterial leading to rapid reduction of inflammatory lesions.

Benzoyl peroxide is formulated in a number of concentrations ranging from 2.5 percent to 10 percent. In general, one should start therapy with the lowest concentration. The major side effects encountered with this product are excessive dryness, irritation, and allergic reactions. As these untoward reactions increase with higher concentrations, and several studies have failed to demonstrate significantly improved efficacy with higher dosing, most individuals are best maintained on lower strengths. Individuals with sensitive skin may not be able to tolerate this compound, and it should be noted that benzoyl peroxide will stain clothing.

Over-the-counter formulations containing benzoyl peroxide include ProActiv, Clean and Clear and Oxy. In 2014 the FDA issued a warning that certain OTC products containing benzoyl peroxide can induce "rare but serious and potentially life-threatening" allergic reactions and advised that "these serious hypersensitivity reactions differ from the local skin irritation that may occur at the product application site, such as redness, burning, dryness, itching, peeling, or slight swelling, that are already included in the drug facts labels." The same warning was issued for products containing salicylic acid, also used to treat acne. If such reactions do indeed occur their incidence is extraordinarily uncommon given the tens of millions of consumers that have safely used these ingredients for decades.

Benzoyl peroxide is a potent oxidizing agent that kills germs on contact. Unlike with antibiotics, bacteria do not develop resistance to this agent. Prescription benzoyl peroxide may be combined with the topical antibiotic clindamycin (Acanya, Benzaclin, Duac, Onexton) or a topical retinoid (Epiduo).

Sulfur

Sulfur-containing compounds have been used to treat acne since the 1800s. Sulfur has anti-inflammatory activity, and many formulations have a distinctive odor. Some sulfur-based products are available over the counter (for example, Rezamid), while others require a prescription (i.e. Avar, Klaron, and Sulfacet-R).

Retinoids

Another modality commonly used to treat acne consists of the topical application of vitamin A derivatives called retinoids (examples include Atralin, Differin, Retin-A, and Tazorac). These substances possess comedolytic properties; they dislodge dried sebum and help keep the pores open. There is increasing evidence that retinoids may also exert a direct anti-inflammatory effect upon the follicle. The major downside of such therapy is undue irritation.

Most vitamin A derivatives utilized as acne therapy require a doctor's prescription. Undesirable side effects include facial redness, peeling, and burning. These reactions frequently diminish with repeated use.

Skin treated with retinoids may become very sensitive to sunlight and easily sunburned. For this reason, excess sun exposure should be minimized. In fact, at least in the summer months, prescription retinoids are best applied only at night and thoroughly washed off in the morning.

Antibiotics

The topical antibiotic clindamycin is available in solution, gel, and foam formulations (i.e. Cleocin-T, Clindagel, Evoclin). Azelaic acid (Azelex, Finacea) is an antibacterial cream derived from wheat. Dapsone gel (Aczone) is latest topical antibiotic approved as acne therapy; interestingly, the oral form is used to treat leprosy.

As mentioned, a topical antibiotic may be combined with benzoyl peroxide therapy to decrease the potential for bacterial resistance. Clindamycin is also effective when combined with a retinoid (Veltin, Ziana).

Oral antibiotics are the mainstay of therapy for moderate to severe acne. As a general rule, antibiotic treatment for this condition begins with a tetracycline derivative such as doxycycline (i.e. Acticlate and Doryx) or minocycline (i.e. Minocin and Solodyne). Oral tetracyclines have been used to treat acne for decades and these drugs have an admirable safety record. The lowest dose of an antibiotic necessary to control acne is a prudent course of action, with discontinuation recommended once adequate control is achieved.

Tetracycline derivatives are best not taken with milk or vitamin-mineral combinations because these substances lessen GI absorption. They should not be administered to pregnant or nursing women as well as to children under the age of eight as teeth staining in the neonate or child will result.

Minocycline in high doses may produce dizziness (vertigo) and has been linked to blood chemistry abnormalities and skin pigmentation. Doxycycline may uncommonly cause sun photosensitivity. Gastrointestinal side effects may be minimized by taking these medications with food.

Contraceptives

Although some oral contraceptives may aggravate acne, others may reduce oil production and promote acne clearing. Women with persistent acne who do not respond to more traditional therapies may be candidates for such hormonal manipulation. Certain birth control pills (Ortho Tri-Cyclen, Estrostep, and Yaz) have been approved by the FDA to treat acne. The drug spironolactone helps counteract the male hormone and may also prove useful for women with moderately severe breakouts.

Isotretinoin

In 1982 a powerful medication for the treatment of severe acne was released in the United States. Called isotretinoin (trade-named Accutane), this "miracle" drug has revolutionized acne therapy.

Isotretinoin is a derivative of vitamin A and is available in capsule form. The medicine is generally administered for a five- to six-month period. Within three weeks of commencing the medication, varying degrees of skin dryness may occur at times accompanied by dry eyes, cracked lips, and nosebleeds. These somewhat annoying side effects often last for the duration of therapy and tend to be most severe with higher dosing. Isotretinoin may also raise the level of circulating fats, and for this reason periodic blood tests are mandatory.

For those with cystic acne, the results of isotretinoin therapy are well worth any transient aggravation. The disfiguring cysts resolve, and for the majority of people completing treatment, new cysts rarely appear. Some 80 percent of such patients achieve long-lasting remission. By preventing deep cysts, isotretinoin abruptly halts the dreaded sequela of acne, scar formation. Some individuals with persistent yet less severe forms of acne may benefit as well.

Controversy exists regarding the association of isotretinoin with mood changes, depression and colitis; direct links, if they do occur, are certainly rare. Regarding the latter, trial lawyers had a field day suing manufactures for alleged causation of inflammatory bowel disease (IBD). A large population-based study published in 2014 concluded that isotretinoin use was not associated with this condition; in fact, this medication may even protect against one form of IBD, Crohn's disease.

Isotretinoin must *never* be taken by pregnant women because of the high incidence of birth defects. Women of childbearing age must practice strict birth control. Isotretinoin should only be administered under a dermatologist's care. Indeed, persons on this drug must be registered in a central government-mandated database called I-Pledge. Isotretinoin is available under the trade names Amnesteem, Claravis, Myorisan, Sotret and Zenatane. The drug is best taken with a meal to enhance absorption. Absorica is a unique form of isotretinoin that demonstrates superior absorption to the others when taken without food. Daily doses of isotretinoin range from 10 mg to 80 mg. Factors used to determine individual dosing include body weight, severity of acne, and incidence and extent of undesirable effects such as excess dryness.

Other Treatments

What about the physical methods used to treat acne? Again, please remember not to pop pimples or further manipulate acne lesions unless properly instructed by a dermatologist. Extraction of open comedones (blackheads) can be accomplished under proper supervision by use of a comedone extractor. This instrument features an open loop that is placed over the blackened pore, allowing the contents to be expressed when firm pressure is applied. Comedone expression has minimal influence on the course of acne. The widened pore will reaccumulate its blackened contents within a month's time; however, many persons obtain cosmetic and psychological benefit from this procedure and welcome the removal of these unsightly black dots.

Most recently, lasers, IPL (intense pulsed light), blue and red light sources, and even a topically applied solution activated by light have been employed as acne therapies. Such interventions, of varying costs, may lessen the need for oral antibiotics. The verdict is still out as to the overall effectiveness of these physical modalities, which are somewhat expensive and generally not covered by health insurance.

Persons who develop large, disfiguring cysts benefit from the injection of a steroid solution (Kenalog) directly into each cyst. This medicine often dramatically reduces the size of a lesion within twenty-four hours and may prevent subsequent scarring.

Scarring

What can be done for those already scarred by acne? Dermatologists and plastic surgeons possess several tools for the correction of scarring, including dermal filler implants, dermabrasion (mechanical sanding), and lasers. Which procedure(s) to use depends on a number of factors, including the extent and depth of scarring. Shallow, concave, pliable scars respond immediately to dermal filler injection. In 2015 the FDA approved the dermal volumizer Bellafill as a scar correctant. Superficial scars may respond to multiple laser sessions. Satisfactory results are being reported with fractional laser photothermolysis and a procedure called needling which entails needle sticks into the dermis to stimulate collagen. Consult with a dermatologist who is knowledgeable in all facets of scar correction. Keep in mind that although 100 percent correction is unlikely, some degree of improvement may be achieved. Often the changes are dramatic.

In summary, the immediate goal of acne therapy is to clear up existing pimples and blemishes and prevent new ones from appearing. Mild acne may respond to topical therapy with over-the-counter preparations containing benzoyl peroxide, sulfur derivatives, or salicylic acid. However, if these measures fail, an appointment with a dermatologist is prudent. The skin care specialist has at his/her disposal a variety of beneficial treatments for acne. Two or more different medications are commonly employed at the same time. One must bear in mind that such regimens rarely produce instant results; acne does not clear up overnight. Be patient! You should always give a new regimen a minimum of three to four weeks for visible results to occur.

Those with cystic acne that is unresponsive to antibiotics are strongly advised to consider isotretinoin. Certain scars may improve with injectable fillers or laser therapy.

Acne is a cosmetically disfiguring problem. If left untreated, the condition may lead to immense physical and emotional scarring. Today acne is certainly controllable, and select cases may be cured.

ROSACEA AND PERIORAL DERMATITIS

Rosacea and perioral dermatitis are two facial disorders that affect women in greater frequency than men. Both are striking causes of a red face.

Rosacea

Rosacea begins very insidiously, often as a prominent, evanescent facial flush. The rosy condition may involve only the lower half of the nose or may spread to cover the "blush zone" comprising the cheeks, forehead, and chin. The bouts of redness gradually become more frequent and intense, leading to persistent changes in skin color. The end result is permanent facial redness along with numerous enlarged blood vessels. Rosacea may be accompanied by crops of inflamed pus-filled pimples.

According to the National Rosacea Society, the condition affects over fourteen million Americans. Over 75 percent of patients responding to an annual survey admitted that rosacea lowered their self-confidence and self-esteem. Rosacea usually occurs in middle-aged women, those between ages thirty and fifty-five. The condition seems to affect people who, since childhood, have blushed easily, as well as those who develop intense redness following only brief sun exposure. The most severe form of rosacea affects men and afflicts the nose. Medically termed rhinophyma, the disorder is characterized by uneven, progressive nasal swelling (the "W. C. Fields nose") and may cause significant cosmetic deformity.

Rosacea may also affect the eyes (ocular rosacea). Individuals so afflicted may experience itching, stinging, dryness, foreign body sensation, and a watery, bloodshot appearance.

The exact cause of rosacea is unknown and treatment often proves difficult. The condition is aggravated by the ingestion of hot beverages and alcohol, both of which dilate blood vessels and promote facial redness. Extremes in temperature, as well as excessive sunlight, should be avoided. Several studies implicate overgrowth of a harmless microscopic facial mite (called Demodex) in the pathogenesis of rosacea.

ROSACEA TRIGGER FACTORS	
Sun exposure	Vigorous exercise
Stress	Wind
Alcohol	Hot baths
Caffeine	Cold weather
Spicy foods	Hot beverages

Persons with rosacea should avoid harsh cleansers, toners, and astringents. When outdoors broad-spectrum sunscreen application is highly recommended. The mainstay of the medical treatment for rosacea is the oral antibiotic doxycycline, which often must be taken for years. Trade names include Acticlate, Doryx and Oracea, the latter a low-dose version promoted specifically for rosacea. Topical preparations containing the antibiotic metronidazole (Metrogel, Noritate) may prove useful in both the treatment of acute flares and long-term maintenance, as may sulfur-containing compounds (Avar, Klaron, Sulfacet-R), and medications containing azelaic acid (Azelex, Finacea). In 2014 the topical cream Soolantra (1% ivermectin) was approved to treat rosacea; this medication reduces colonization of the Demodex mite.

The best way to cover up the redness associated with rosacea is to apply a green tinted foundation or concealer underneath one that is skin-toned. The prescription medications Mirvaso gel (brimonidine) and Rhofade (oxymetazoline) are approved to treat rosacea-associated facial redness. When applied daily these medications result in significant, albeit temporary, redness reduction although not all people respond and a small percentage experience side effects such as skin irritation. The treatment of choice for the dilated blood vessels accompanying rosacea is either specific vascular lasers (i.e. the V-Beam) or IPL (intense pulsed light). Both are simple office procedures with the primary downside of temporary bruising. Results are quite rewarding. Some patients remain clear following a single session whereas others require treatment two to three times per year. Insurance companies do not cover light therapies as they are considered cosmetic in nature.

Perioral Dermatitis

Perioral dermatitis is a facial condition that primarily affects women in the twenty- to forty-year age group. Over the past decade, the problem has become increasingly more common.

The development of tiny red pimples and pustules, as well as dryness and scaling around the mouth and on the chin, characterizes perioral dermatitis. Occasional burning or itching may be experienced.

Perioral dermatitis may last from several weeks to many years. The condition waxes and wanes in intensity, and premenstrual worsening is common. The use of high-potency steroid creams will either cause or exacerbate this facial rash, and such use must be immediately discontinued. Medications containing sulfur (Avar, Klaron, and Sulfacet-R) often afford adequate control, although some cases may require oral antibiotic therapy.

PERSPIRATION

Virtually all humans perspire and each year American consumers spend some 750 million dollars on underarm products designed to inhibit sweating and prevent offensive odor. Perspiration occurs over the entire body, but it is most abundant in the underarm and genital areas owing to the large accumulation of sweat glands at these sites. Newly formed sweat is acted on by bacteria to produce the characteristic body odor known to every kid as "B.O." A deodorant either masks this odor or decreases its production by inhibiting some of the underarm bacteria. Antiperspirants, on the other hand, act by reducing the flow of glandular perspiration. Commonly used antiperspirants frequently contain aluminum compounds that inhibit sweat production.

Antiperspirants and deodorants are marketed in a variety of forms including creams, roll-ons, and aerosols. The first two are more efficient and cost-effective, the latter more convenient. With the increasing concern over personal health and the environment, the use of certain aerosols has been curtailed.

Antiperspirants and deodorants are generally safe and effective. If mild burning or irritation develops, one would do best to switch to another brand. Baking soda (sodium bicarbonate) works quite well, and those with sensitive skin might consider use of this inexpensive, readily available compound.

Excessive Perspiration: Hyperhidrosis

It is of course normal to sweat, but some of us are plagued with an exaggerated sweat response. Called hyperhidrosis, this distressing condition may affect the palms and soles, as well as underarm areas. Profuse sweating results from even the least amount of heat, or physical or mental activity. Emotional stress may also trigger hyperhidrosis. The hands, feet, and underarms produce a steady stream of moisture ("sweating buckets") leading to marked self-consciousness in most hyperhidrosis sufferers. Survey data suggests that over one million Americans are negatively impacted by excess sweating.

Hyperhidrosis often begins during puberty and improves with age. Topical therapy with a nonprescription "clinical strength" or "extra strength" antiperspirant should be the first line of therapy. Examples include Certain Dri, Secret Clinical Strength, Dove Invisible Solid, and Degree Invisible Solid. The ideal time for application is at bedtime, as these agents work best when applied to dry skin. Persons not achieving adequate control should try a prescription antiperspirant such as Drysol. These solutions contain aluminum chloride in strengths ranging from 15 to 20 percent. Again, nighttime application to dry skin is crucial for success. A deodorant may be applied in the morning for cosmetic purpose.

Iontophoresis therapy (also called drionics) uses a battery-powered device intended to inhibit excess sweating of the hands, feet, and underarms. The small current induces electrical charges in the sweat glands that decrease sweat production. The treatment is safe but relief is variable, and therapy has to be continued indefinitely. Oral medications such as Ditropan, Robinul, and Probanthine may prove extremely helpful and are quite safe; higher doses may induce the annoying side effect of a dry mouth. The MiraDry system is a microwave energy device used to treat axillary hyperhidrosis through selective heating of the lower layer of skin, where the sweat glands are located. The treatment results in irreversible loss of these glands. Cost is significant and side effects are common, including post-treatment swelling, redness and discomfort in the treatment area although most patients are said to be pleased with the end result.

Botox, injected into the underarms, palms and soles (and even into the face and scalp), is a simple method to alleviate hyperhidrosis. Approved in 2004 by the FDA for use in excessive sweating of the underarms, Botox is now considered the gold standard of therapy. Drawbacks include transient discomfort during injection (multiple sticks are required) as well as high cost (usually not covered by insurance) and limited duration. Injections need to be repeated every six to nine months. The vast majority of individuals treated with Botox express satisfaction with this procedure. Both Dysport and Xeomin, also neurotoxins administered by needle, produce similar results

Surgical excision or liposuction may be utilized to remove sweat glands situated within the armpits. A more drastic option is surgical destruction of the nerves that control sweat production (sympathectomy), a procedure usually performed under general anesthesia, which is generally reserved for physically or psychologically incapacitating sweating.

ITCHY SKIN

Itching (medically termed pruritus) is a sensation that produces a desire to scratch. Itching may be localized to a specific area (for example, the site of a mosquito bite), or it may be generalized over the entire skin surface. People respond to an itch in different ways, the response in large part depending upon the personality of the affected individual. A mosquito bite, for example, may be violently scratched until it bleeds, gently rubbed, or simply ignored.

A wide range of factors can produce itching. These include inflammations of the skin caused by external irritants such as harsh soaps, infections (especially those caused by yeast and fungi), infestations such as scabies and lice, allergic reactions including contact dermatitis and hives, and specific skin disorders such as eczema.

On occasion generalized itchiness may be associated with certain abnormal systemic conditions. Diabetes, liver disease, kidney failure, and even cancer are at times accompanied by diffuse itching. Itchy skin may also occur during pregnancy.

A very common cause of itching is dry skin (xerosis). Too frequent bathing with hot water and strong soaps, advancing age, and cold weather all contribute to skin dryness. The legs are the most commonly involved sites. The condition may be improved through the use of moisturizing creams and bath oils.

One of the most important sources of itching is psychological, that is, a reaction to stress and strain. An anxious male tends to scratch his scrotum, whereas an uptight female frequently concentrates on the back of her neck.

People suffering from mental illness (psychosis) may become convinced that their skin has been invaded by parasites. These deluded individuals pick and dig until sores develop, and they are obviously in dire need of psychiatric care.

Anal itching (pruritus ani) is a very common, annoying problem. The condition may be engendered by numerous factors including anxiety and nervous tension, hemorrhoids, contact with irritating chemicals and soaps, parasites (crabs, lice, and pinworms), and fungal and yeast infections. Circumstances that worsen the itching include excess perspiration, obesity, tight clothing, frequent bowel movements, inadequate cleansing, and occupations that require long periods of sitting (for example, truck driving, office work).

Several general measures may provide total or partial relief of pruritus ani. Cleansing after each bowel movement should be particularly thorough, using only minimal amounts of a mild, non-medicated soap. All soap must be completely rinsed off the area after cleansing. Moistened facial tissue, rather than ordinary toilet tissue, causes less irritation. Prolonged sitting (during long car trips, for example), tight clothing, and overstuffed chairs should be avoided. A daily sitz bath and frequent applications of an occlusive paste such as zinc oxide ointment may prove beneficial. Cases of pruritus ani not responding to these measures should be evaluated by a dermatologist, gynecologist, or proctologist.

Itching can be a very distressing symptom. Any itch is made worse by wool clothing, friction, excess warmth and sweating, reduction of body oils by frequent washing, and the use of harsh soaps. Inactivity and relaxation tend to make one more aware of an itch (hence itching is usually most severe at night).

A self-limited itch, such as an insect bite or a mild case of poison ivy, may be lessened by cool compresses and/or application of an over-the-counter anti-itch preparation such as Itch-X or TriCalm or the prescription medication, Alevycin. Persons with itching associated with visible skin lesions such as solid bumps or water blisters may require consultation with a dermatologist. Those who have persistent, generalized itching with no apparent skin disorder may require a medical examination and laboratory testing to rule out a serious underlying medical condition.

HAIR, SCALP AND NAILS

Normal Hair

The scalp contains approximately one hundred thousand hairs. Each hair attains a maximum length and then enters a resting stage, following which, it falls out. Unlike certain animals, which shed their entire outer layers at once, humans have hairs that act independently; normal human hair loss occurs in random fashion and is quite inconspicuous. Some one hundred scalp hairs are regularly shed on a daily basis (This may seem like a large number, but it represents only one-thousandth of the total scalp hair).

Hair grows at different rates depending on its location. Scalp hair expands at a rate of one-hundredth of an inch per day; in other words, one hundred feet of new hair is manufactured on a daily basis. Each scalp hair is capable of growing for three to ten years. This is in contrast to the hair of the armpits and eyebrows, which has a growth period of less than 1 year; these hairs grow to fixed lengths and then enter into a prolonged resting period.

The hair that we look at, fondle, and spend so much time and money on is merely dead tissue. Living hair is produced from protein under the skin within a structure called the hair follicle. The hair is no longer alive by the time it reaches the surface.

Each follicle is attached to an oil gland and is surrounded by nerves and muscles. The muscles are very sensitive to cold and contract on stimulation, pulling the hair follicle and wrinkling the skin surface. This action gives rise to the tiny raised pimples known as goose bumps.

Hair differs in both amount and consistency among the various races. Whites are the hairiest, followed by blacks, with Asians being the least hirsute. Asians have the straightest hair, while blacks have the curliest.

Hair color depends on the number of pigment cells (melanin) within the hair shaft. Blond hair contains few pigment cells, and the snow-white hair of the elderly has virtually none. Red hair is due to an iron-bearing pigment.

Gray Hair

As we age, so does our hair. Aged hair is grey or white. To date, despite advertising claims touting melatonin, copper blockers, and vitamins, the only effective treatment is hair dye. But there is hope. Some of the aged follicles from which hair grows still contain miniscule amounts of pigment cells, and recent evidence points to a buildup of hydrogen peroxide in older follicles which prevents these cells from producing pigment (melanin). Finding a way to decrease hydrogen peroxide within the follicle may reverse the graying process.

Reports periodically surface that hair-coloring agents promote cancer. Fortunately, this does not appear to be the case, and if there is a risk, it is quite minimal. Hair dyes can however trigger allergic reactions, hence the warning on package inserts to test the skin prior to each application. Allergic reactions do appear to be on the rise as more, and younger, individuals dye their hair. The main culprit is an ingredient called paraphenylenediamine (PPD). An allergy to hair dye may result in an itchy, red rash of the scalp, ears, and face, at times accompanied by swelling.

Damaged Hair: Split Ends

Since the hair visible to us is dead, and since it is constantly growing from under the scalp, any damage that occurs to hair above the skin is fortunately temporary. Hair problems caused by the environment and improper treatment will improve, given time and correct management.

Our hair suffers from an incredible amount of physical and chemical abuse. The longer the hair, the greater the extent of this trauma. Those of us with hair two feet long have ends nearly three years old! Over this time period, just imagine the amount of brushing, combing, pulling, curling, setting, shampooing, hot-air drying and sun, salt, and chlorinated-water exposure this hair has been subjected to. Small wonder some of us have split ends!

Split ends (the frizzies) are the result of excessive trauma to hair. The problem is usually more severe in longer hair. When performed in moderation, combing, brushing, and blow-drying do not damage hair. When such activities are too frequently and vigorously undertaken, however, split ends are the inevitable result. (Researchers can manufacture split ends in clipped normal hair by utilizing a hair-rubbing apparatus.) Blow-drying is safe as long as it does not continue after the hair is dry to the touch; over-drying leads to fragile, easily damaged hair. Similarly, chemical treatments such as bleaching, waving or curling, and straightening may damage hair under certain circumstances.

Damage to hair may be lessened by use of conditioners and cream rinses. These compounds coat the hair surface and reduce combing friction. They may also guard against some of the deleterious effects on hair from blow-drying and sun exposure. The only cure for split ends once they occur is cutting them off; avoidance of excessive damage, coupled with the judicious use of conditioners and cream rinses, will minimize their occurrence.

Hair Loss: Pattern Alopecia

As we have noted, an insignificant amount of hair is lost from the scalp on a daily basis. On occasion, hair is shed at such a rapid rate that the loss does indeed become noticeable. Such hair loss may either be generalized or confined to distinct areas.

Male pattern baldness is a hereditary disorder that first becomes apparent in late adolescence or early adulthood. Progressive hair loss is noted in the front and center of the scalp and is due to the slow shrinkage and subsequent death of hair follicles.

Millions of dollars' worth of quack tonics and megavitamin pills "guaranteed" to reverse the hair-loss process and grow hair are sold annually. Advertised in popular journals or on late-night TV shows, many of these products prey on men's vanity and as a rule disappear following state or federal investigations. Some meld science with pseudoscience, referencing DHT (dihydrotestosterone, a known causative factor of male pattern baldness) and concoctions of poorly studied herbal remedies.

To date, only two products are FDA approved to retard or reverse male pattern alopecia: minoxidil (Rogaine) and finasteride (Propecia). A third, dutesteride (Avodart) has demonstrated efficacy in clinical trials.

Minoxidil (in pill form) was first marketed as an oral treatment for high blood pressure. Problems soon became evident when the drug was administered to women and children: they began to sprout beards and mustaches!

A true genius got the bright idea of rubbing the stuff on the shiny scalps of bald men, and—lo and behold—new hairs indeed began to grow. This was indeed a monumental accomplishment, the first time in history that something grew new hairs. It is known that minoxidil dilates blood vessels, but the mechanism of action on scalp hairs is still unclear.

Minoxidil does not work on everyone. People with the least amount of hair loss, and those balding for the shortest time period, appear to do best. For many of these individuals, minoxidil results in significant hair growth. For the majority, minoxidil will help prevent or delay further thinning of the hair. By starting minoxidil treatment early, male pattern baldness may be placed on hold. The trade name for minoxidil is Rogaine, now available in both liquid and foam formulations.

Finasteride (Propecia) is used in higher doses to treat an enlarged prostate. This oral medication was approved in 1997 as a treatment for male pattern baldness. The drug inhibits the breakdown of the male hormone, testosterone, to DHT. Clinical studies demonstrate that finasteride can induce new hair growth in about 50 percent of men and can also increase the weight and diameter of existing hair. As is the case with minoxidil, therapy with finasteride is for life; once discontinued, the natural process of hair loss will proceed. Finasteride's long-term effect on general health is unknown; however, data indicates that chronic use may actually decrease the risk of prostate cancer, a very significant finding.

Dutasteride (Avodart) acts in a similar manner to finasteride but has a longer half-life. In other words, two pills per week may keep a guy's hair intact. And, on another positive note, a study published in 2009 concluded that Avodart lowered the risk of prostate cancer by 23 percent.

For those unaided by, or deciding against use of either minoxidil or oral agents, depleted hair may be covered up by a toupee or hair weave, or partially rectified by hair transplantation.

Hair transplant traditionally involved the transfer of quarter-inch round plugs from the back of the scalp to thinned areas in the front of the scalp. The technique was analogous to placing sod down on a depleted lawn and results in permanent replacement. The cosmetic endpoint varied from natural to comical, with many individual heads resembling cobblestone roads. Nowadays, follicular unit transplantation has supplanted plugs; it involves removing thin strips of hair from the posterior scalp, which are then dissected into thousands of micro-grafts prior to transplantation. The results are much more natural and, in many people, virtually imperceptible.

Some physicians are utilizing lasers in attempts to slow down hair loss and stimulate new hair growth. Indeed, units are now available for home use. Until adequate clinical studies are published, laser use for baldness should be viewed with a healthy degree of skepticism. The same can be said for platelet-rich plasma injections administered under the scalp.

Generalized hair loss in women may occur as a result of certain stressful situations. For example, increased hair shedding frequently follows pregnancy. The loss of hair may be mild or quite marked and can occur from the first to twelfth week after delivery. No treatment is necessary as the hair completely grows back. Such hair loss is called telogen effluvium.

Women taking birth control pills may experience diffuse hair thinning, either while on these pills or shortly following their discontinuation. Again, this hair loss is only temporary and fully corrects itself within a few months.

Classic female pattern hair loss is also called androgenetic alopecia. The condition most commonly occurs around menopause and characteristically involves the front and top of the scalp. Treatment with minoxidil may stabilize the condition. Rogaine for women is now available in a 5 percent concentration which is superior to the traditionally used 2 percent formulation. Users should take care to apply minoxidil only to the scalp and let it thoroughly dry before resting the head on a pillow to avoid unwanted facial hair. Minoxidil should not be used by pregnant or nursing females. The oral medication spironolactone helps to block male hormone uptake by the hair follicle, although clinical response is slow. Minigraft hair transplantation is another option for women and may yield excellent cosmetic result. Use of finasteride and dutesteride in post-menopausal women with hair loss has been advocated by some dermatologists.

Want fuller eyelashes? In 2009 the prescription eyelash-enhancer Latisse became available. Applied like eyeliner, Latisse enters eyelash hair follicles and results in longer, thicker, and darker eyelashes. Not cheap, but works.

Hair Loss: Alopecia Areata

A common form of localized hair loss that occurs in males and females, and in children as well as adults, is alopecia areata. In this condition a circular zone of complete hair loss rapidly develops, leaving the scalp smooth and shiny. The affected area may range from dime-sized to larger than a silver dollar. Multiple patches may occur.

The cause of alopecia areata is unknown, although an abnormality of the immune system is suspected. Some cases follow emotional stress and tension. Most of the hairless patches spontaneously grow hair in two to three months. Very rarely, the hair loss may become generalized leading to severe cosmetic disability, especially in women. Dermatologists treat localized forms of this disorder with steroid creams and/or injections.

Hair Loss: Traumatic

Some neurotic or psychotic persons consciously or subconsciously pull at and twist their hair until breakage occurs. This compulsive behavior is called trichotillomania and results in patchy zones of hair loss within which are found broken hairs of uneven length. Chronic cases warrant psychiatric consultation.

Various cosmetic manipulations can lead to hair loss. Traction produced by tight rollers or braids may so weaken the hair as it exits the scalp that patchy areas of reversible baldness result. The kinky hair of blacks is particularly prone to fracture. Such traction alopecia is most noticeable on the sides of the scalp.

Bleaching, setting, and permanent wave solutions will not significantly damage hair unless applied in an inappropriately high concentration or over a prolonged time. However, the frequent use of hot combs and oils to straighten hair (a cultural adaptation practiced by many African Americans) may cause marked scarring of the scalp and permanent baldness. "Hot-comb alopecia" most commonly occurs in the center of the scalp.

Several "hairy" myths must be debunked here as well. The plucking of hair does not produce permanent baldness (nor does it cause the hair to grow in thicker). Cutting, shaving, or massaging the scalp has no effect on hair growth. Frequent hair washing and shampooing also do not lead to hair loss, nor does dandruff (no matter how severe).

Excess Hair

Excess hair growth is known as hirsutism. For most individuals, the problem is simply a cosmetic one, indicating neither the presence of hormonal nor of gender abnormalities. In fact, if one examined a group of white females, nearly one-quarter would be found to have hair on the upper lip (with the condition being very apparent in 10 percent), and over three-quarters would exhibit coarse hair on their arms and legs.

Hair distribution is in large part genetically determined; if your mother has excess facial hair, you most likely will too. In general, women of southern Mediterranean and Near Eastern origin have more facial and body hair than do North American and Asian women.

About 1 percent of women complaining of excess body hair have a significant medical problem such as overactive adrenal glands or ovaries. Such women may also experience menstrual irregularities, weight gain, and acne. Since both benign and malignant tumors must be ruled out, hirsute women with these associated disorders should visit a physician and undergo examination and laboratory studies. Some drugs, such as Depo-Provera, Dilantin, and tamoxifen, can also induce hirsutism.

Many women are quite concerned about excess body and facial hair. Several means are available for the removal of unwanted hairs, the current gold standard being lasers and intense pulsed light (IPL).

Lasers and IPL are specialized light sources. Light used for hair removal passes through the skin and is absorbed by pigment within the hair follicle. The procedure can be safely performed on virtually any part of the body with excess hair, except about the eyes. Hair that is coarse and dark responds best to laser treatment. Blond, white or red hair is difficult to treat. As the pulses of light energy are of brief duration, discomfort is momentary.

Laser and IPL hair removal usually require multiple sessions, and in most cases, the results are best referred to as reduction rather than permanent removal. Approximately 20 to 30 percent reduction will be noted after each treatment with long-term hair reduction approaching ninety percent. Treatments are repeated every four to six weeks depending on location (shorter time intervals are required for hairs above the neck). Note that the FDA allows approved manufacturers to claim "permanent reduction" but not "permanent removal" for their devices.

Side effects associated with laser and IPL hair removal are transient redness, inflammation of the hair follicles (folliculitis), activation of fever blisters, pigmentary changes, and (rarely) scarring.

Commercially available light-based hair reduction devices for home use are now available. These appear to be safe and somewhat effective, although determining just how effective will require larger studies. Make sure that any light or laser device marketed for hair reduction is approved by the FDA before using it but note that FDA approval does not equate to efficacy.

Unsightly hair may be removed by electrolysis. In this procedure a tiny needle is placed within each hair follicle and a short burst of current is administered. The electrical charge destroys the follicle and prevents further hair growth. Similar to lasers and IPL, multiple treatment sessions are required.

Electrolysis is time-consuming, somewhat painful, and not inexpensive. Results range from acceptable to excellent. Electrolysis is a viable alternative to treat light-blond, white, and gray hairs, as these are not amenable to light-based treatment modalities.

Shaving with either a safety razor or electric shaver is a simple, temporary means of hair removal. As noted, repeated shaving or plucking with a tweezers does not lead to increased or thickened hair growth. Hair plucking pulls the hair from the root. Results last about six weeks.

Another means of hair removal consists of the application of depilatory creams. These compounds cause a transient dissolution of surface hair following a brief application time ranging from five to ten minutes. Their use on sensitive skin may produce irritation.

Objectionable hairs may be rendered inconspicuous through bleaching. Again this is a simple, albeit temporary, measure to lessen the unfavorable cosmetic impact of excess facial hair.

Vaniqa is the first FDA-approved prescription cream utilized to slow the growth of unwanted facial hair in females. About half of women who use this product, applied twice daily, experience satisfactory hair reduction after several months of therapy. Hair excess linked to ovarian dysfunction is often treated with birth control pills.

Dandruff: Seborrheic Dermatitis

The medical term for dandruff is seborrheic dermatitis. This condition tends to affect hair-bearing regions and facial furrows; it is not a disorder of hair but of the underlying skin. Seborrhea literally means "freely flowing sebum," and the problem occurs in those areas with a large number of oil glands. Common sites include the scalp, eyebrows, central face, external ear, mid chest, upper back, belly button, and genital areas.

The most common form of seborrhea consists of slight redness coupled with an itchy, greasy, scaling dandruff, with white flecks that rain down on dark-colored clothing. Seborrheic dermatitis may become more severe, producing bright-red, inflamed, scaling patches on the face and chest that may spread under the arms and even to the groin.

No cure exists for seborrhea, but in most cases, the disorder is easily controlled. Seborrheic areas are very sensitive and readily irritated. Scratching and rubbing the skin only serves to prolong the condition and may lead to infection. People with excess oil and scaling of the scalp must shampoo regularly. A shampoo especially formulated to control dandruff should be used at least twice weekly. Active ingredients in dandruff shampoos include selenium sulfide (Head & Shoulders Selenium, Selsun Blue), zinc pyrithione (Denorex Daily Protection, DHS Zinc, Head & Shoulders), tars (Denorex, DHS Tar, Neutrogena T/Gel, Pentrax, Tarsum), ketoconazole (Nizoral), ciclopirox (Loprox), and topical steroids (Clobex). The latter two are available only by prescription.

To be effective, a dandruff shampoo should remain on the scalp for at least five to ten minutes before rinsing. Over time, a shampoo may lose effectiveness. Should this occur, the best course of action is to switch to another type of shampoo. Those with a more severe form of seborrhea may require cortisone in the form of a gel, foam, spray, or lotion prescribed by a physician.

Nails

Our nails are made of keratin, a rock-hard, shiny substance. As is the case with hair, the nail itself is dead. The living part of the nail lies under the skin in a region called the matrix, and it is here that new keratin is formed. Thus, any physical damage that we inflict on the outer nail is temporary, for new keratin is constantly being produced by the matrix. Fingernails grow at a rate of one-eighth of an inch per month, toenails even slower. If a fingernail is lost, about six months are required for a new one to completely grow back. Regrowth of a toenail might take nearly one and a half years. Damage to the matrix, on the other hand, may lead to gross distortion and permanent loss of the affected nail.

Deformities of the nail may be caused by trauma, fungal infections, and by certain diseases such as psoriasis. Nail discoloration is often due to physical factors; a black nail results from injury, a yellow nail from cigarette smoking. Greenish nails may be caused by a pigment-secreting bacterium (genus *Pseudomonas*). The tiny white flecks that adorn so many nails are probably produced by minor insults such as excess nail filing or nail biting. Sometimes nail changes indicate serious internal disease. Clubbed nails may be a sign of lung cancer; spoon-shaped nails, a sign of anemia. The bed of the fingernails should be light pink. White nail beds may indicate anemia. Nails that are white and opaque may be a sign of liver disease whereas half-and-half nails (bottom white, top pink) may point to kidney disease. Although a black nail is usually the result of trauma, you should be careful; sometimes pigment under a nail is a consequence of malignant melanoma, the most deadly form of skin cancer.

Nails, like hair, are made of protein. Similarly, nail strength and texture may be adversely affected by nutritional deficiencies but will not be improved by the ingestion of excess protein, calcium, or yeast. The notion that gelatin will enhance nail growth and luster is simply a myth.

Many women complain of brittle nails. This distressing but harmless condition appears to be caused by microscopic loss of water from the keratin. Some women derive benefit by soaking the affected nails in lukewarm water and then coating each nail with a moisturizing ointment. Several small studies support the use of the B vitamin biotin as a treatment for brittle nails.

Fingernail length is a matter of personal preference. Because toenails are subjected to weight bearing and close confinement, their length should be regulated by proper trimming. Each toenail should be "squared off" when cut, not clipped too deeply where the sides of the nail are in contact with the skin. Improper cutting of toenails as well as ill-fitting footwear and improper gait can lead to ingrown toenails, a troublesome condition that may require minor surgical correction by a podiatrist or dermatologist.

Applying polish to nails is a safe procedure that has no effect on nail health and growth. Very rarely a woman may develop an allergy to nail polish, characterized by redness and itching wherever the substance comes in contact with skin. A woman runs a far greater risk of becoming allergic to those compounds used in nail sculpturing, and for this reason, many have been taken off the market. Acrylic nails cause little harm, unless left on for too long. Best practice is to remove them at least once every three months and to allow two to three weeks prior to reapplication.

Swelling at the base of a nail is called paronychia; the affected area is red and tender. Paronychias of longstanding duration are seen almost exclusively in women. Until recently the underlying cause was thought to be yeast infection, but more recent evidence suggests that chronic environmental stress (repeat contact with detergents, solvents, or the like) is the most likely culprit. Treatment involves keeping the nail as dry as possible, using a topical steroid cream or gel, and when indicated, undergoing topical or oral anti-yeast therapy.

One of the most common nail problems is fungal infection. Fungal infections of the nails begin at the free margins and sides and result in yellowish discoloration, increased thickness, and marked fragility. Toenails are more frequently affected than fingernails.

Because of the distortion and color changes, nail fungal infections are often an embarrassment. This problem is difficult to treat effectively and oral therapy offers the best chance of cure or extended remission. Terbinafine (Lamasil) is now considered the drug of choice and, despite the meteoric rise in the cost of drugs, remains quite affordable and has a good safety record. Three topical formulations in solution form, all FDA-approved to treat fungal nails, are Jublia, Kerydin and Penlac. These should be applied to affected nails on a daily basis over many months. Lasers are currently in vogue and heavily advertised. Therapy is expensive and results are questionable to date. On occasion, individuals opt for surgical or chemical removal of the infected nails, but there is no guarantee that the new nail will be free of infection.

CELLULITE, STRETCH MARKS AND FAT REDUCTION

Cellulite is a cosmetic nuisance of great concern to millions of American and European women. The condition has engendered a number of nonmedical books and articles on the subject, as well as a billion-dollar industry that is in the habit of proclaiming that cellulite can be simply "melted away." Laypersons who treat cellulite with a variety of creams and mechanical devices are doing a thriving business in a growing number of spas.

Cellulite is not a disease but the result of a naturally occurring process that affects the thighs and buttocks of many women as they age. With the passage of time, the fat cells in these areas become less organized and lax, giving rise to the lumps and depressions so characteristic of cellulite. Cellulite is not associated with physical discomfort; the only pain is psychological. Men are not affected because of the lesser amount of fat (adipose tissue) in the locations where cellulite typically forms.

Two factors contribute to the appearance of cellulite: heredity and obesity. If your mother has cellulite, chances are good that you will too. Your risk of cellulite appears to be enhanced if you are overweight and out of shape.

No magical cure exists to reverse the pits and depressions of cellulite. A variety of enzyme injections (mesotherapy), special diets, and external suction devices are currently being used by estheticians for this purpose. Scientific studies documenting efficacy are lacking.

Persons with cellulite are advised to lose weight and exercise. Some middle-aged women have experienced an improvement in their condition with careful weight reduction. Crash dieting is to be avoided because the drastic loss of weight will actually worsen the cosmetic appearance. Regular exercise and massage (stroking the skin with the hand or a brush) may also prove beneficial. Do not be deceived by the incredible "cures" so heavily promoted in women's journals.

Use of a pressure devise (a procedure called endodermatology) as well as application of creams containing aminophylline may improve some cases of cellulite, as may liposuction. However, results are disappointingly short-lived and liposuction may actually cause worsening in some cases.

A device called VelaSmooth combines infrared light, radiofrequency, suction, and massage. This device is claimed to "loosen the fat-collagen bands under the skin and firm up the top layers of the skin." SmoothShapes combines laser and light along with suction and massage "to treat the causes of cellulite by restoring the adipose cells and improving the fibrotic fibrous septae." Studies to date show modest improvement in some patients, but the duration of benefit, when noticeable, remains in doubt. A *Wall Street Journal* article on the subject offered this summary: "the latest cellulite treatments sound too smooth to be true."

Stretch marks, medically termed striae distensae, are a form of scar tissue that affects the dermal layer. They initially appear as pink, reddened, or purplish lesions that over time whiten. Affected areas include the breasts, abdomen, hips, thighs, buttocks, and upper arms.

Stretch marks are most commonly associated with pregnancy, developing to some degree in approximately 75 percent of women prior to delivery. Contributing factors include weight gain and hormonal changes. Stretch marks can also occur in men, especially those who rapidly gained muscle mass as a consequence of weightlifting with or without illicit steroids.

Prevention is difficult. Avoidance of rapid weight gain or loss is prudent. Steroids taken to gain muscle mass are potentially dangerous and may induce not only striae but more serious medical conditions as well. Pregnant women may benefit from a combination of moisturizers and massage.

Treatment of stretch marks is best undertaken at an early stage when the lesions are discolored. Indeed, a goal of therapy is to hasten the conversion of reddened or purplish patches to lighter, less visible hues and 1% hydrocortisone is worth a try. How well specific over-the-counter topicals such as Mederma Stretch Marks Therapy work is open to conjecture although supported by anecdotal accounts.

Retinoids such as Retin-A (tretinoin) promote production of collagen and can improve stretch marks. Several studies document improvement following laser, IPL, and fractional photothermolysis. These therapies reduce the redness associated with early striae and may increase skin elasticity, as may the procedure micro-needling. Multiple treatment sessions are usually required.

The procedure called tumescent liposuction, as opposed to traditional liposuction, is performed in the specialists office under local anesthesia. Once numb, a thin hollow tube is inserted and excess fat is suctioned out. Discomfort and swelling may last several days. Bruising is common and resolves within two weeks. Maximum results may take several months to attain and these may last for years. Tumescent liposuction is commonly used to reduce the belly and love handles, slim hips, and reshape the jawline and neck.

Noninvasive procedures to reduce fat are gaining in popularity although the results are usually less dramatic than those achieved with liposuction. Application of cold to the skin helps dissolve fat cells, a procedure called cryolipolysis or coolsculpting. Multiple sessions are required for maximal result but downtime is minimal.

In 2015 the FDA approved the injectable medication Kybella to treat excess fat under the chin, The best candidates are individuals with a mild to moderate amount of fat and good skin elasticity. Each session entails multiple injections (up to 50) and several sessions, scheduled no less than 1 month apart, are usually required. The most common side effect is bruising.

DILATED BLOOD VESSELS

Telangectasias

Minute dilated blood vessels (enlarged capillaries) are known medically as telangectasias. They appear as thin, red strands (called "spiders") that often lose their color upon application of pressure. Since the vessels are permanently dilated, the color promptly returns when the pressure is removed.

Most telangectasias are found on the face, but they may also occur on the chest and back. "Spiders" are frequently encountered in perfectly normal persons, especially those with fair skin. They increase in number with age and with excessive sun exposure. Pregnant women may develop multiple telangiectasias, as may persons suffering from chronic alcoholism and liver disease. One of the hallmarks of rosacea is the appearance of facial telangiectasias.

Spiders are harmless, but they often pose a cosmetic nuisance. A single lesion can be treated in the dermatologist's office with a tiny needle through which is passed a momentary electric current. Multiple lesions are best treated by laser (such as the V-beam), a virtually painless and very effective procedure. A transient bruise is the only adverse event.

Cherry Angiomas

Cherry angiomas are bright red dots that appear on the skin surface and are commonly found in individuals after the age of forty. The most common location is the trunk. Cherry angiomas are composed of thin blood vessels which first appear as pinpoint dots and gradually enlarge, at times reaching the size of a pencil eraser. They are painless and harmless but cosmetically unappealing. If traumatized, profuse bleeding will result. The lesions can be removed quite simply by either electrocautery or a laser.

Leg Veins

As a person ages, blood vessels (venules) within the calves and thighs expand in diameter. Varicose veins are larger vessels that range in color from flesh-toned to dark blue and often have a bulging, cord-like appearance. Spider veins are smaller in size and closer to the surface. Often they network in a pattern similar to a tree branch. Hereditary predisposition, obesity, prolonged standing, hormonal changes, and pregnancy are contributory factors, and over 50 percent of women are affected.

Spider veins have no medical significance but are unsightly. The most common treatment is called sclerotherapy; it entails injection of the offending vessels with a sclerosing agent administered through a tiny needle. The procedure is accomplished without local anesthesia, and discomfort is usually momentary and minimal. When performed by an experienced health care provider, complications are infrequent and not serious; at times bruising may result, but this gradually fades. Common sclerosing agents include sodium tetradecyl sulfate, polidocanol, and hypertonic saline (concentrated salt solution). Following injection, a compression bandage should be applied for twenty-four hours. A successful injection produces dissolution of the dilated vessel over a three- to six-week period.

Laser therapy is a more costly solution and works best on those vessels of tiniest diameter. Minute bursts of intense light are directed into the veins, and when the procedure is successful, fading gradually ensues. Although somewhat painful, laser treatment appeals to some individuals because it allows them to avoid needles and injections. Often two to five treatments are required for adequate cosmetic result. As with sclerotherapy, there is no downtime.

Varicose veins can be a sign of venous insufficiency. At times they may ache. Workup entails physical examination and at times ultrasound analysis. Sclerotherapy may be effective. The treated vein frequently shows signs of inflammation and clotting, both of which are not serious and respond to hot compresses.

Larger vessels may be surgically removed by phlebectomy or stripping with ligation. These procedures are best performed in a surgi-center or hospital and entail small excisions followed by dissection of the offending vessels.

A more recently developed therapy, called endovenous ablation, entails the insertion of a catheter that emits radiofrequency energy into the vein.

Alternatively, laser light can be administered using a fiber. The end result is shrinkage of the vein wall.

Bear in mind that a key to the prevention or recurrence of leg veins is compression. For predisposed individuals, graduated support compression stockings are recommended for use during daytime hours.

AGING AND THE SKIN

The skin is no different from any organ in the body; it too ages. But unlike other organs, aging skin is visible to us and to others.

Young skin is characteristically taut, smooth, and evenly pigmented. Skin that is old has become thin, discolored, lax, and wrinkled. As skin ages, several distinct changes occur. Aged skin suffers from fluid depletion. The water-holding capacity diminishes, and the oil-secreting glands dry up. This results in a marked propensity toward dryness and chapping. Old skin frequently features prominent scaling.

Physiologic functions of skin include barrier protection, temperature regulation, sweat production, sensation perception, and production of vitamin D. By middle age, many of these functions are reduced, some by as much as 50 percent or more. Senile skin is characterized by a thinning out of the outermost layer, the epidermis. In some elderly persons, the skin becomes so atrophic that it resembles cigarette paper.

The layers under the epidermis (that is, the dermis and the subcutaneous tissues) also decrease in thickness. Tiny fibers that support the skin lose their springiness; if one stretches an older person's skin, it does not "bounce back" into its original position as would a young person's. As skin matures, collagen becomes fragmented, and new production is reduced. The combination of tissue loss coupled with loss of elasticity results in the hallmark of aged skin, wrinkles.

Aged skin is more susceptible to a variety of disorders and diseases than normal skin. Because of the lack of moisture, senile skin has a tendency to dry out, this being especially severe in low humidity. As skin dries it becomes chapped, cracked, and intensely itchy. The more aged the skin, the greater the number of dilated and broken blood vessels, which is a cosmetic nuisance. Skin cancer occurs at an increased rate with each passing year. Besides the cosmetic disfigurement, this problem poses a real threat to general health.

Three main factors are known to contribute to skin aging: heredity, sunlight, and smoking.

Much of the aging process is genetically determined, something programmed into an individual's body even before birth. This is also termed intrinsic or chronological aging. If your parents have young-looking skin, chances are good that, barring physical abuse, you will too. Unfortunately, the contrary also holds true. The skin of some individuals seems to age at an accelerated rate no matter how much it is pampered.

The rare condition called progeria is characterized by premature aging of all organs, including the skin. Children with this disease have wrinkled, aged skin, comparable to the skin of an elderly individual. Werner syndrome is a condition that appears similar and strikes individuals in their late teens. The genetic defects responsible for both disorders have been uncovered, and it is hoped that these findings will shed additional light on the normal aging process.

The sun is a bitter enemy of healthy skin. Repeated, prolonged exposure to sunlight leads to irreversible premature aging, called photoaging. Ultraviolet light stimulates formation of free radicals that damage DNA within epidermal cells and decrease the amount of collagen in the dermis. Some degree of this aging can be anticipated with each prolonged exposure. Excessive sunlight leads to thinned and yellowed skin, broken blood vessels, brownish discolorations (liver spots), and skin cancer.

Some idea of the injurious effects of sunlight can be gleaned by examining the skin of a person who has spent a great deal of time outdoors. Look closely at the face of a career fisherman or sailor. His skin will be dry, cracked, and wrinkled; and he will appear much older than he actually is, because his skin has aged prematurely.

If you are a person who has spent much time in sunlight, compare the skin of your face and hands to that of your lower breast and buttocks. The areas exposed to chronic sun are apt to be discolored, rough, and wrinkled. That beautiful tan of yesteryear has long ago faded, leaving in its wake damaged, unhealthy skin.

Several studies document that cigarette smoking also leads to premature aging of the skin. One study compared identical twins; the skin of the twins who smoked was 25 percent thinner than that of the twins who did not. On a molecular level, cigarette smoke activates the genes responsible for a skin enzyme that breaks down collagen.

The term *smoker's face* was coined over two decades ago by a physician who was able to differentiate smokers from nonsmokers, not by the soot and carcinogens clogging their lungs, but by facial features alone. The smoker's face is characterized by accelerated skin aging, deep wrinkles about the mouth, and accentuated crow's feet. Even secondhand smoke is absorbed into and through the skin.

Regarding premature aging, we cannot alter our genes. But we can in large measure control exposure to sunlight and cigarette smoke.

Dermatological Treatment of the Aging Face

Few people enjoy the aging process, especially when it involves our skin. Given that we cannot literally turn back the hands of time, what can we do to reverse the ravages of aging?

Topical Anti-Aging Compounds

Two prescription drugs may be used to combat the aging process: Renova (identical to Retin-A, which is used to treat acne) and Avage (identical to Tazorac, also used to treat acne). Both are FDA approved for use in the mitigation of fine wrinkles, mottled hyperpigmentation, and tactile roughness of facial skin in patients who use comprehensive skin care and sunlight avoidance programs. In other words, both products are used to improve (and possibly prevent) fine wrinkles, smooth skin, and lighten dark spots in conjunction with protection from solar radiation. Both do work, albeit slowly. Used on a long-term basis, Renova and Avage may actually prevent a certain degree of wrinkling. (Note: neither will work on deeper wrinkles or creases)

When applying Renova or Avage, use only a miniscule amount to avoid undue dryness and irritation. A pea-sized amount is enough to cover the entire face. A good regimen is to apply a moisturizer with a sunscreen in the morning, and the prescription anti-aging medication at night.

A number of nonprescription skin creams are widely available and heavily promoted. "Active" ingredients include retinol (a form of vitamin A), various peptides, resveratrol, and alpha hydroxyl acids. A Consumer Reports 2012 clinical study of nine facial antiaging serums, ranging in price from $20 to $65, concluded that: "after six weeks of use, the effectiveness of even the best products was limited and varied from subject to subject." As most individuals use anti-aging formulations on a chronic basis, comparison over a longer time period would be of greater value.

Microneedling

Microneedling is a minimally invasive procedure that uses a device with fine needles to puncture the skin. The end result is production of collagen and elastin, substances that add firmness to the skin and contribute to texture. Discomfort is minimal and areas treated are reddened for up to three days. Several treatments are recommended at intervals ranging from three to six weeks followed by yearly maintenance. Although home units are available, these are not as effective as in-office devices and pose a risk for infection.

Chemical Peels

Chemical peels have been used to rejuvenate facial skin for decades. Peeling involves the application of an exfoliating and/or wounding agent to the surface of the skin. Depth of penetration and degrees of exfoliation and skin sloughing are dependent on a number of factors, the most important being the actual chemical used for the peel. Other factors may include concentration of the peeling agent and time left on the skin surface.

A light peel stimulates epidermal rejuvenation by gently removing the stratum corneum. A medium-depth peel causes partial destruction of the epidermis and induces inflammation. Deep peels are uncommonly utilized because of the risk of scarring and pigment alteration.

Superficial peels are used to improve the tone and texture of skin. The most commonly used peeling agents are glycolic and salicylic acid. Side effects are uncommon.

Medium-depth peeling agents include Jessner's solution, glycolic acid, and low to medium concentrations of trichloroacetic acid. These may even texture and tone, lighten dark spots, and diminish fine lines secondary to sun damage. Redness is to be expected, but this fades over a seven- to ten-day period. Complications include untoward pigmentary changes (especially in people with dark skin), reactivation of fever blisters, and (rarely) scarring. Chemical peels may be combined with laser resurfacing for facial rejuvenation.

Botox/Dysport/Xeomin

Botox, approved for cosmetic use in 2002, is now the most widely utilized cosmetic procedure in the United States with millions of injections administered each year. The simplicity of administration, rapidity of results, lack of serious side effects, and high degree of satisfaction has combined to revolutionize the field of minimally invasive aesthetic procedures.

Botox is a toxin produced by bacteria. Injected in dilute amounts it results in temporary paralysis of superficial muscles. The drug is FDA approved for the temporary correction of forehead frown lines and wrinkles about the eyes (crow's feet). Botox is administered through a tiny needle; the entire procedure takes minutes and entails minimal discomfort. Desirable results are obliteration of unsightly, age-related lines within hours to days after injection. The effect lasts four months on average. Off-label, Botox is used about the mouth and even on neck muscles, but the results in these locations are variable.

Side effects of Botox are uncommon and include headache and eyelid drooping. The latter, medically termed ptosis, is a temporary but disconcerting nuisance that may last anywhere from a few days to a few weeks.

The cost of Botox varies. Some providers (doctors, nurse practitioners, physician assistants) charge based on areas treated, others by the amount (units) administered. One vial of Botox (one hundred units) costs the provider hundreds of dollars. Equally efficacious as Botox are two other competing neurotoxins: Dysport and Xeomin.

In 2009 the FDA added a black box warning of possible serious side effects related to use of neurotoxins. Given the millions of injections and the rarity of adverse events, it appears that serious reactions have only occurred as a result of off-label use for certain chronic disease states, not for the treatment of wrinkles and lines. Nevertheless, finding a well-trained, experienced health care provider to administer the neurotoxin is always a wise decision.

Dermal Fillers

Although Botox is very effective in minimizing forehead lines and crow's feet, it cannot restore fullness, particularly to the lower face, lost as a consequence of the aging process. Indeed, volume loss is one of the hallmarks of an aging face and dermal fillers are ideally suited for this purpose.

The first dermal fillers approved by the FDA were Zyderm and Zyplast. Introduced over two decades ago, these injectable compounds revolutionized the treatment of lines and creases. Zyderm and Zyplast were made from bovine (cow) collagen. Collagen, of course, is one of the foundations of the dermis. Both products were short lived and could trigger allergic reactions necessitating allergy testing prior to use.

Fat transplantation was developed as one way of bypassing the need for allergy testing, since the fat injected under a crease was derived from fat cells taken from the same individual (abdomen or backside). A major drawback was longevity as the transplanted cells would disappear within a few months. New techniques have resulted in greater survivability of the fat cells.

The dermal filler market exploded in 2003 with FDA approval of Restylane. Restylane is non-animal-derived hyaluronic acid; this a normal component of the body substance that surrounds skin cells. Prior allergy testing is not required, allowing for same-day administration. Additional FDA-approved hyaluronic acid fillers include Belotero, Juvederm, Perlane, and Prevelle Silk. Results last for several months to over a year. Side effects are uncommon and include redness, bruising and persistent bumps. Repeated injections may stimulate the natural production of collagen.

Radiesse is a filler composed of calcium. This product has no allergic potential, and the correction often lasts eight months or longer. Radiesse has been demonstrated to both augment collagen and stimulate production of new collagen as well. Sculptra, which consists of poly-L-lactic acid, is not a conventional replacement filler. Small amounts are injected over time, and the end result is stimulation of collagen. Visible results are gradual and develop over weeks. Bellafill is an injectable collagen filler with microspheres that provides both immediate and longer term correction. Juvederm Voluma contains cross-linked hyaluronic acid and provides greater longevity than other hyaluronic acid products.

As a rule, the longer a filler lasts, the more careful (and experienced) a provider should be in administering it. The choice of filler often depends on the area to be treated.

Nasolabial folds (the two creases running from the nose to the corners of the mouth) and marionette lines (creases from the mouth corners to the chin) are amenable to the majority of fillers. Factors to consider are price, longevity, and the experience and preference of the medical provider performing the injections. Lip augmentation requires a less viscous filler to avoid the complication of persistent bumps. Corrections about the eye entail minute amounts of a thinner filler, whereas depressions of the mid-cheek region are best handled with a thicker volumizer or dermal stimulator.

Laser Rejuvenation

Laser resurfacing is characterized as either ablative or nonablative. Ablative resurfacing entails wounding of the skin surface. Lasers for this purpose are the CO2 and erbium:YAG varieties. During the ablative process the epidermis and parts of the dermis are removed resulting in improvement of skin texture, uneven pigmentation, and some correction of wrinkles. Downtime is significant, with marked redness and crusting lasting at least ten days. Scarring is possible, and the procedure is best not performed on more darkly pigmented individuals. Fractional ablative lasers break light into thousands of microbeams that bore tiny holes in the epidermis. The result is skin tightening of variable degree with less downtime. Healing occurs within six to ten days.

With nonablative resurfacing, the beam of laser light passes through the epidermis and stimulates new collagen production in the dermis. Downtime is nil with minimal redness. The results are often subtle and may not become apparent for weeks to months. A series of treatments are required approximately four to eight weeks apart. Periodic touch-ups are recommended.

Intense pulsed light (IPL) uses non-laser light to improve pigmentation, reduce unsightly blood vessels, and even smooth texture. This too is a nonablative technique.

With the latest technique, nonablative fractional resurfacing, the laser creates so-called micro-thermal zones of controlled skin damage. Mildly photodamaged skin usually improves with this technique, but deeper wrinkles do not.

Anti-aging is big business. Looking one's best can often be accomplished with minimal discomfort and virtually no downtime. The use of neurotoxins, dermal fillers and volumizers, microneedling, and lasers will continue to soar.

THE SUN AND SKIN

We are a society accustomed to sun worship with bronzed skin a symbol of leisure and good health. Soaking up rays is often a favorite pastime and come nightfall a glance in the mirror reveals the payoff of a day's "work," the suntan.

WARNING: Sun Exposure May Be Hazardous to Your Health!

Many of us express deep concern regarding the hazards of nuclear power, yet think nothing of basking all day in solar radiation. We have learned that the sun's ultraviolet rays damage the skin's elastic tissues, leading to unsightly skin lines and wrinkles. The end result is premature aging and, for some, skin cancer. Each year, over two million cases of skin cancer are detected in the United States, where one person dies from skin cancer every hour. Ultraviolet light is responsible for the majority of skin cancers.

Besides the long-term effects attributed to chronic sun exposure, the damage wrought by sunlight may become apparent much sooner. Acute overexposure results in the painful, all-too-familiar sunburn.

SUNBURN

Virtually every light-skinned person has experienced sunburn at one time or another. Sunburn is a discomforting condition most frequently encountered at the beginning of summer before a protective tan has been acquired. Redheads and blonds burn readily; dark-skinned persons may sunburn, but only after prolonged exposure to strong sunlight. A recent study of fifteen thousand adults found that one-third had experienced a sunburn within the past year.

The extent of sunburn may range from a mild, painless redness to a fiery red, exquisitely tender, blistering eruption. A mild burn begins some six to twelve hours from the beginning of exposure, reaches a maximum redness within twenty-four hours, and gradually declines over the next few days, leaving in its wake tanned skin that may take some two weeks to reach its peak.

Severe sunburn also begins six to twelve hours following sun exposure, but within one to two days marked skin changes occur. The skin becomes extremely painful to even the slightest sensation. Chills, fever, and nausea are commonplace. Fluid-filled blisters appear, and layers of the skin begin to slough off. Uneven pigmentation and even scarring may result.

Mild sunburn reactions may be treated with cool water compresses. Emollient creams can soothe the skin and relieve dryness. Over-the-counter burn preparations contain local anesthetics that may help alleviate discomfort but will not enhance healing. Aspirin controls the pain and may even lessen the inflammation.

Severe sunburn should be treated by a physician. Cortisone pills and antibiotic creams are sometimes necessary to limit the inflammation and prevent infection.

SUN PROTECTION: How to Remain Safe in the Sun

Some dermatologists urge the avoidance of all nonessential sunlight whenever possible. Sun tanning is frowned upon. Other dermatologists are a bit more lenient and the risks versus benefits of sun exposure are hotly contested in the scientific literature.

Six different skin types are defined. The lower your skin type number, the greater the risk of developing significant damage from exposure to sunlight or indoor tanning.

Skin Type	Sunburn & Tanning Traits
I. Sensitive	Always burns easily; never tans
II. Sensitive	Always burns easily; tans minimally
III. Normal	Burns moderately; tans gradually

IV. Normal	Burns minimally; always tans well
V. Insensitive	Rarely burns; tans profusely
VI. Insensitive	Never burns; deeply pigmented

The sunlight that reaches the earth consists of visible light and ultraviolet (UV) radiation; the invisible ultraviolet rays cause suntans and sun-induced skin injuries. The amount of ultraviolet light reaching the skin depends on a number of factors. For example, the lower the latitude, the greater the risk of sun damage to the skin at any given hour. A noontime sunbather in Miami will experience a heavier dose of burning rays than a noontime sunbather in Boston. The time of greatest risk anywhere in the world occurs in the middle of summer between the hours of 10 AM and 2 PM.

Seasonal variations and altitude also play a role in the amount of ultraviolet light striking the skin. One will experience a more severe suntan in early May than at the end of August. The higher the altitude, the less atmosphere is present to filter out ultraviolet rays, a contributing factor to the marked sunburns often seen in winter skiers.

Environmental factors may also enhance one's chances of sunburn. Beach sand, snow, and shiny metal (as in sun reflectors) markedly increase the dose of solar radiation. Other factors may fail to offer adequate protection. Water is not an efficient sun blocker; burning and tanning rays can penetrate beneath the surface of a pool. Many people sunburn on overcast days. Fooled by the lack of visible light, they do not take adequate protection, unaware that invisible ultraviolet radiation still reaches the skin. In fact, 70 percent of the sun's rays penetrate clouds and fog.

Potentially harmful ultraviolet radiation is divided into UVA and UVB. UVA constitutes over 90 percent of the radiation penetrating to the earth's surface. UVA can also penetrate the skin's surface and has been implicated in suppression of the immune system and causation of skin cancer. UVB causes damage to the epidermis, this resulting in the acute sunburn. Chronic ultraviolet light exposure induces wrinkles and other signs of cutaneous aging. UVB is filtered by window glass, but UVA is not.

A first line of defense against untoward ultraviolet light exposure is clothing, with some garments being much more effective than others. Indeed, certain clothes, especially when wet, fail to protect the skin from a significant portion of ultraviolet light. Color (darker shades being more efficient), fiber content, and fabric weave help determine clothing's effectiveness as a barrier to ultraviolet light.

Individuals who are extremely sun sensitive or those who are at high risk for skin cancer would do best to wear specially formulated protective clothing when sun avoidance is not possible. Manufacturers include Coolibar and Solumbra. Another option is to wash clothes using the laundry additive Rit SunGuard which confers adequate UV light protection that lasts for about twenty washes.

And don't forget a hat, especially if your hair is thinning. The hat protects not only the scalp, but depending on brim size, parts of the face as well.

Sun protective agents applied to the skin are known as sunscreens. These are widely available, formulated as creams, gels, lotions, sticks, pads, and sprays. Some ingredients work best to block UVA and have esoteric names such as avobenzone (Parsol 1789) and terephthalydene dicamphor sulfonic acid (Mexoryl SX). Others block UVB and have unpronounceable names such as octyl dimethyl para-aminobenzoic acid (PABA) and ethylhexyl p-methoxycinnamate. Agents that block both UVA and UVB are referred to as inorganic sunscreens and contain titanium dioxide or zinc oxide.

Since both the ultraviolet A and ultraviolet B spectrums of light are dangerous to skin, one should always apply a sunscreen labeled "broad spectrum."

For maximum effectiveness, sunscreens should be applied thirty minutes before sun exposure and reapplied after swimming or profuse sweating. A "water resistant" sunscreen will adhere to the skin while the user is in water for forty minutes. A "very water resistant" sunscreen will adhere for eighty minutes. As a rule, most sunscreens lose their effectiveness after three or four hours.

The amount of sunscreen used is an important factor. One ounce (two tablespoons) is the minimal amount needed to cover the entire body. According to a study in the *British Journal of Dermatology* most people only apply one-quarter of the amount of sunscreen that they should.

Concerned about the growing incidence of sun-induced skin problems, as well as undocumented claims by certain manufacturers, the U.S. Food and Drug Administration advised in 1978 that sun protection factor (SPF) information be included on all sunscreen packages. Sunscreen products now carry numbers ranging from 15 to 50+ indicating their effectiveness in filtering out solar radiation capable of burning the skin. The higher the SPF number, the greater the degree of protection from UVB.

The SPF number provides a convenient way to calculate how long an individual can stay out in the sun without burning. Suppose that, with no tan at all, you can normally stay out in the sun ten minutes before getting burned. If you now use a product with an SPF of 15, you can stay out in the sun 150 minutes (10 X 15) without burning.

The higher the SPF number, the greater the shielding from burning radiation. This is not a linear relationship; an SPF of 30 does not give twice as much sun protection as an SPF of 15. SPF 15 blocks 93 percent of burning rays; SPF 30 blocks 97 percent; and SPF 50 blocks all but 1 percent. In 2013 the FDA mandated that any product with an SPF lower than 15 must carry a label warning that it will not protect against skin cancer. The FDA also questions the merit of using any sunscreen labelled above 50

Remember, SPF refers *only* to UVB radiation protection. Maximum sunscreen protection is afforded by a *high-SPF*, *broad-spectrum* formulation. This is important because UVA radiation has been linked to premature aging and skin cancer. And again, applying the correct amount of sunscreen is crucial. Using half of the correct amount of sunscreen rated at SPF 50 (that is, one tablespoon rather than two) will not give a SPF of 25, but one of 8.

If used properly, sunscreens will prevent the immediate danger from solar radiation, the sunburn. Long-term use will help prevent wrinkles, dark spots, and cancer. Because the hazardous effects of sunlight are cumulative, sunscreens are best used at an early age.

Kids and Sunscreen

Sunscreens of any type are not recommended for children younger than six months; regardless of age, small tots are best physically shielded from direct sunlight. The FDA is currently investigating the use of spray-on sunscreens due to the risk of particle inhalation and exacerbation of asthma or allergic reactions; as of this writing children (and possibly adults as well) should not use sprays. Several sunscreens are specifically marketed for children and these contain ingredients less likely to irritate the skin such as titanium dioxide and zinc oxide.

Indoor Tanning

The Food and Drug Administration and the American Academy of Dermatology are concerned about health hazards posed by indoor tanning centers. You should be too. Sunbed ultraviolet light emission is ten times more potent than natural sunlight. Most of the radiation received in tanning booths is ultraviolet A, linked to skin cancers and cataracts. Because of these risks, the majority of states have enacted age restrictions regarding light box tanning and over one-fifth of states now prohibit the use of indoor tanning booths by minors. In 2014 the FDA mandated that all indoor tanning devices carry warning labels. Still, some thirty million Americans are expected to tan indoors annually. In 2013, about 20 percent of high school girls and 5 percent of high school boys had sought out some form of indoor tanning at least once in the previous year.

Melanoma is the second most common cancer among American women in their twenties, and the rate of new melanoma cases in younger women has soared, increasing by 50 percent since 1980. Women under thirty-five who use sunbeds increase their risk of developing melanoma by an astounding 74 percent. Melanoma has the potential to kill.

The Department of Health and Human Services and the World Health Organization have deemed ultraviolet light a known carcinogen (cancer-promoting agent). The number of skin cancer cases due to indoor tanning is higher than the number of lung cancer cases due to smoking.

A 2015 review in the Journal of the American Academy of Dermatology offers an apt summary: "Evidence demonstrates unequivocally that tanning beds cause sunburn, photoaging, development of skin cancer, and full addictive behaviors while supplying no scientifically supported health benefits".

TANOREXIA

The concept that UV tanning is addictive has gained ground over the past several years, and the condition has been given the name *tanorexia*. Studies have demonstrated that frequent tanners experience withdrawal symptoms when UV tanning is abruptly discontinued. A study that recruited college students found that 12 percent of those interviewed showed evidence of a UV light-substance-related disorder. Despite awareness of the dangers of tanning, many still believe that tanner people are better-looking.

SELF-TANNERS

Scores of self-tanning formulations are available on the market for those seeking to *look* tan. The first self-tanning product was introduced way back in 1960, Coppertone QT (Quick Tanning) lotion. The problem? Rather than look golden brown, users tended to resemble aged pumpkins. Fortunately, shades are now quite realistic and pleasing. This fact, coupled with increased public awareness of the dangers of ultraviolet light, have contributed to the soaring popularity of these products.

The most effective sunless tanning gels, lotions, and sprays contain an ingredient called dihydroxyacetone (DHA), a colorless sugar that stains the cells in the top layer of the epidermis. DHA is the only agent currently approved by the FDA for this purpose. Stained cells are already dead and slough off in about five to seven days, hence the need for reapplication. Most commercial products contain a mixture of DHA, bronzers (water-soluble dyes that temporarily stain skin), and moisturizers. DHA does appear to be safe long-term when used on the skin surface, with low incidence of allergic reactions. Keep in mind that most products containing DHA offer no—or, at best, inadequate—sun protection, and that stained skin remains vulnerable to ultraviolet damage.

Tan accelerators are said to lessen the exposure time needed to bronze skin. Many contain the amino acid tyrosine, and all require ultraviolet light for activation. The FDA is "not aware of any data demonstrating that tyrosine or its derivatives are effective in stimulating the production of melanin." (Stimulation of melanin is what produces a suntan.)

Oral "tanning pills" typically contain the substance canthaxanthin, which is FDA approved as a food-coloring agent. In high quantities the compound is deposited in the skin. But it is also deposited in the liver and eyes and can lead to hepatitis and cataracts. Canthaxanthin as a tanning agent is now banned in the United States but is available via the Internet.

SAD

No doubt, when the sun doesn't shine, many of us become depressed. This is termed SAD (seasonal affective disorder), and the features are depression, lack of energy, and an increased need for sleep. The mildest form is known by most as "winter blues." About 75 percent of those affected are women, and the most common age of onset is in the mid-thirties. SAD is believed to affect fifteen million Americans, and perhaps another thirty million display some symptoms. The treatment of choice is bright light—the visible kind—not ultraviolet. And the light does no good striking the skin; it must be visualized by the eye.

True, SAD may be treated in the middle of winter in NYC with a bright white light source, but one can surmise that, if given as an option, Florida beach therapy would get the nod hands (if not buns) down. If you are lucky enough to fulfill this option, remember—especially if you are fair-skinned or have a personal or family history of skin cancer—to protect body parts from dangerous ultraviolet rays.

More on Vitamin D

Vitamin D helps the body absorb calcium and maintain adequate levels of calcium in the blood stream; both tasks are necessary for maintaining healthy bones. Vitamin D deficiency can lead to bone diseases, including osteoporosis. Vitamin D is the most commonly supplemented vitamin, added to milk, bread, and orange juice. Sun or exposure to ultraviolet light of the B range induces skin cells to manufacture vitamin D. The amount produced depends on a number of factors including exposure time, altitude, latitude, extent of skin surface exposed, time of year, and skin pigmentation (the darker or more tanned the skin, the less produced). Use of a high-SPF sunscreen limits the skin from forming vitamin D.

Some clinicians have suggested that higher levels of vitamin D may protect against prostate, colorectal, and breast cancers, and can help prevent heart disease as well as improve fatigue and muscle weakness. Unfortunately, the majority of evidence to date does not support any of these claims.

Vitamin D levels can be measured, and medically supervised oral supplementation will correct deficiency. Studies suggest that relatively small amounts of sun exposure, ten to fifteen minutes on sunscreen-free hands, face, and arms two to three times a week, are sufficient to maintain adequate levels. So, a little sun may go a long way.

Yes, a little sun. Millions of dollars each year are spent on topical formulations and procedures to prevent or reverse the ravages of aging. Yet a major factor that contributes to the aging process is sun and ultraviolet light exposure. Certainly many individuals can tolerate varying degrees of sun exposure, especially those with darker skin. Others cannot. Individuals of skin type I (persons with very pale skin, blue eyes, blond or red hair) and skin type II (persons with fair skin) experience skin damage with each and every exposure. Keep smoking cigarettes, and chances are good that you will develop lung cancer or emphysema. Keep chasing that golden tan, and the day may soon arrive when that taut, bronzed, "healthy" covering gives rise to a shriveled, discolored, cancer-infested prune.

BENIGN SKIN GROWTHS

Benign growths are those skin lesions that are not cancerous (malignant). They may be annoying from a cosmetic standpoint, but as a rule they do not endanger one's overall health.

Skin Tags

Skin tags are tiny, soft, fleshy outgrowths of skin that usually have an onset in early to middle adult life. They more frequently occur in women and are found around the neck, upper chest, and armpits. Color ranges from flesh-colored to light brown.

Skin tags cause no discomfort or itching unless irritated. They can be simply removed by carefully snipping them with a pair of manicure scissors. Larger tags are best treated in the doctor's office.

Seborrheic Keratosis

On the beach you may notice that many seniors have darkly colored, seemingly stuck-on growths affecting their skin. These disfiguring lesions are known as seborrheic keratoses.

Seborrheic keratoses are most common after the age of fifty. They are almost always multiple and range in color from yellow to brown to dark black. The surface texture may feel waxy or rough. Common locations are the chest and back, but they may also occur on the face, scalp, and extremities. An individual lesion may attain a size of two or more inches in length, and they can become irritated by friction or trauma.

Seborrheic keratoses are benign skin growths that never become cancers. Although quite unsightly, they fortunately are not dangerous and are readily removed in a dermatologist's office.

Birthmarks and Moles (Nevi)

Birthmarks and moles are lesions composed of specialized pigment cells. A mole may be considered a birthmark that appears on the skin surface later in life. The term "nevus" is applied to both entities.

Nevi are common to all people, and someone searching long and hard enough will find at least twelve or more on most individuals. Some nevi may be present at birth, but the majority arise in young adulthood. It is not uncommon for someone in this age group to have forty or more nevi. A large number of them disappear with advancing age.

Nevi come in a variety of different sizes, shapes, and colors. They range in size from pinpoint specks to extensive lesions that may cover the entire back. (This type of birthmark is fortunately very rare). Their color runs the spectrum from blue to tan to pitch black. Some are perfectly flat, others elevated and dome-shaped. Their surface may be smooth or rough, and some may even have hairs growing out of them.

Many nevi are best left alone. Some occur in areas where they are easily traumatized or cosmetically unacceptable, and these can be removed quite simply. Rarely, a mole may turn into a potentially lethal skin cancer (melanoma), and it is for this reason that nevi should be checked on a periodic basis. The following changes warrant immediate evaluation by a dermatologist:

1. any rapid increase in size;
2. any changes in coloration, especially red or whitish hues;
3. the development of notched, irregular borders;
4. the onset of itching; or
5. the onset of spontaneous bleeding.

All persons with a family history of melanoma or a history of repeated sunburns should have their skin examined on a regular basis.

Warts

Warts are common skin growths caused by a virus. This infection most frequently occurs in children and young adults, and the sites usually affected are the fingers, hands, face, and soles of the feet.

Since warts are produced by a virus, they are contagious. Warts may be spread to different parts of the body as well as to other persons. Many individuals are apparently immune to the virus and are protected from developing warts.

Several different varieties of warts exist:

Common Wart. The common wart is familiar to virtually everyone. This growth appears as a rough-surfaced skin projection (flesh-toned to brown in color) that slowly enlarges in size. The sites most often involved are the hands and fingers. The appearance of one wart may be followed in several months by one, two, or numerous other warts.

Plantar Wart. This wart grows on the bottom of the feet and resembles a callus. It occurs on the weight-bearing areas of the sole and may become quite tender.

Flat Wart. These flesh-colored warts are small, smooth, and slightly raised.

Genital Wart. The genital wart occurs as a moist, pinkish-red growth in the vaginal or anal region or as a firm projection on the shaft of the penis. As with other forms, these growths are spread by close personal contact, in this case by sexual relations. For this reason, genital warts should be considered a sexually transmitted disease (STD). Between five hundred thousand and one million new cases are diagnosed each year.

Warts are certainly a cosmetic bother. Fortunately, about two-thirds disappear without any therapy within two years. Warts are peculiar, as psychological coaxing (for example, hypnotic suggestion) may result in their rapid disappearance. This is probably the reason why folk remedies such as burying a potato under a stump or rubbing a copper penny over the wart did at times cure the condition. Topical, salicylic anti-wart solutions, gels, and patches can be purchased without prescription at any pharmacy. Warts may also be treated in the doctor's office by cryosurgery, electric needle (electrodessication), or laser. Most dermatologists prefer to use liquid nitrogen (cryosurgery) because the procedure is quite effective, can be rapidly performed, and does not involve injection of a local anesthetic. Plantar warts often prove difficult to destroy. Care must be taken to avoid aggressive surgical treatment since painful scarring may result.

Genital warts are treated in the medical office with liquid nitrogen cryosurgery, electrodessication, acid solution, or application of a substance called podophyllin. Both Condylox gel and Aldara cream are approved by the FDA as prescription at-home therapies for genital warts.

Genital warts have been directly linked to the development of cervical cancer, and for this reason women potentially exposed to the causative virus (HPV) are urged to have Pap smears performed on a regular basis. Genital warts also cause anal and penile cancers. More than 40% of adults test positive for HPV exposure. Vaccines that protect against harmful strains of the wart virus are effective and highly recommended for females and males aged 9 to 26. HPV vaccines will actually prevent cancer.

Calluses and Corns

A callus is an area of thickened skin that appears over sites of repeated or prolonged friction and pressure. The involved area is yellow and roughened. Calluses are most commonly located on the palms and serve as a clue to the activity of a person, for example, the callused hands of a bowler or tennis player.

A corn is a discomforting, raised area of skin with a smooth, firm surface that produces pain on pressure. Corns arise most frequently on the top and sides of the fifth toes. Tight, poorly fitting shoes are the usual cause.

Corns and calluses may be treated with acid plaster applied to the lesion and covered with adhesive tape. Painful corns may require surgical removal. Wide, well-fitting shoes prevent the recurrence of most corns.

PREMALIGNANT GROWTHS AND SKIN CANCER

Each year over two million new cases of skin cancer are diagnosed, and the number is steadily increasing. At the present time, skin cancers account for more than half of all malignancies in the United States, and one in six Americans will develop skin cancer in his or her lifetime. Advanced skin cancer can lead to tissue destruction, disfigurement, and even death.

A major contributing factor to the development of skin cancer is excessive sun exposure. Ninety percent of these tumors occur on those parts of the body unprotected from solar radiation; that is, on the face, ears, neck, and hands. Those who have spent a great deal of time outdoors, such as fishermen, sailors, gardeners, and lifeguards, are at greatest risk. The incidence of skin cancer is highest in those areas receiving large amounts of ultraviolet radiation; persons living in Miami or Phoenix have a two to three times greater chance of developing skin cancer than persons living in Chicago or New York.

Heredity too plays a role in the development of skin cancer. Those with fair skin and light eyes (for example, persons of Nordic or British descent) are more susceptible than persons with darker pigmentation (for example, persons of Mediterranean extraction). Persons who redden and blister readily increase their risk of skin cancer with each prolonged exposure to sunlight.

Precancerous Lesions

A precancerous lesion is one that has the potential of becoming a true cancer. Three major types of precancerous lesions exist: solar keratosis, leukoplakia, and Hutchinson's freckle.

Solar Keratosis. Solar keratosis (also called actinic keratosis) is a premalignant lesion caused by the additive effect of long-term sun exposure on the skin. The lesions first appear as flesh-colored to pink, slightly raised, scaling patches located on the face, ears, arms and hands. Solar keratoses are most common in middle-aged and elderly fair-skinned persons. The lesions feel rough to the touch, almost like sandpaper. Unless traumatized or advanced in nature, the lesions are asymptomatic.

Solar keratoses often appear in multiples, and because they do run a risk of turning cancerous, treatment is generally advised. The most common treatment is application of liquid nitrogen, which causes transient stinging. Topical preparations containing the compound fluorouracil (Carac, Efudex, Fluoroplex) can be used to treat larger body surfaces, including the face and arm. Fluorouracil is generally applied daily over a two- to four-week period. During this time, marked redness can be anticipated. Additional topical therapies, all FDA approved for this indication, are diclofenac (Solaraze), imiquimod (Aldara, Zyclara) and ingenol mebutate gel (Picato). Photodynamic therapy, approved in 2000, requires a special light source to activate a topically applied agent. Any lesion that persists despite these therapies is best removed surgically and sent for biopsy to rule out carcinoma. Regular use of sunscreens will reduce the formation of keratoses in predisposed individuals.

Leukoplakia. This condition occurs as discrete white patches that arise on mucous membranes. Areas where leukoplakia may occur include the inside of the mouth, lips, and genitalia. Any thickened, whitish patches at these sites should be evaluated by a doctor.

Hutchinson's Freckle (Lentigo Maligna). This condition occurs most commonly on the cheeks and foreheads of the elderly. It consists of a tan patch that slowly enlarges and darkens. After many years cancer may develop, and for this reason, Hutchinson's freckles are best removed either by surgery or by liquid-nitrogen cryosurgery.

Skin Cancer

Cancer of the skin constitutes the most common form of malignancy. Virtually all skin cancers, if detected and treated early, are curable. Thus it behooves everyone, especially those middle-aged and older, and those who have experienced excessive sun exposure or indoor tanning, to thoroughly check their skin on a regular basis so that any suspicious changes can be immediately brought to the attention of a physician.

Three main types of skin cancer exist:

Basal Cell Carcinoma. Basal cell carcinoma is the most common form of cancer and accounts for nearly 70 percent of all skin cancers. This year well over one million new cases will be diagnosed. Some 99 percent of these cancers occur in Caucasians, especially those with fair skin that burns easily. This tumor usually begins as a small, flesh-colored pimple that slowly enlarges, developing a depressed center surrounded by a smooth, shiny border. Although this type of cancer rarely spreads to organs inside the body, it gradually eats away at the skin and will invade deeper tissues if left untreated. To prevent such destructive effects, these tumors are best removed early in their course.

Squamous Cell Carcinoma. This cancer usually arises in skin damaged by many years of sunlight; that is, in skin that is excessively wrinkled, thinned, and discolored. Sun-exposed areas such as the face, lower lip, neck, and dorsal surface of the hands are the most common sites. Solar (actinic) keratoses and leukoplakia may turn into squamous call carcinoma.

Squamous cell carcinoma frequently occurs as a crusted sore that fails to heal. This malignancy is more serious than basal cell cancer because it can spread internally. Treatment consists of surgical removal or X-ray therapy. Early lesions often resolve with liquid nitrogen cryosurgery.

Malignant Melanoma. Although malignant melanoma accounts for only 3 percent of all cancers of the skin, it produces 65 percent of the deaths from skin cancer. In other words, malignant melanoma is the most uncommon but deadliest form of skin cancer. According to the American Academy of Dermatology, one American dies from skin cancer every sixty-two minutes. The incidence of melanoma has increased 500 percent in the past thirty years, a rate that should alarm us all. According to the Centers for Disease Control, the majority of melanomas are directly tied to ultraviolet light or sunlight, although genetic predisposition plays a role as well. Individuals at highest risk include those with a family history of skin cancer, a history of sunburns as a child, skin that easily freckles and burns, blue or green eye color, blond or red hair, and a large number of moles.

Malignant melanoma may arise on normal skin or from a preexisting birthmark, mole, or Hutchinson's freckle. This skin cancer can afflict persons of all age groups, so anyone with a suspicious new growth or a change in color, size, or contour of an existing mole or birthmark should be examined by a dermatologist as soon as possible.

Everyone should be aware of the ABCDEs of melanoma recognition:

Asymmetry: One side of a mole does not look like the other side.

Border: Irregular or notched borders are a danger sign.

Color: Shades of red, white, or blue may be patriotic, but may also signify skin cancer.

*D*iameter: As a general rule, moles that are smaller than a pencil eraser are okay.

*E*levation or Evolving: Increased height of an existing mole warrants evaluation, as does *any* change.

One can also add the letter I, for itching, as this can be a sign that a mole is transforming into a skin cancer.

And keep in mind the ugly duckling rule as well. Moles on a given individual tend to look alike. The ugly duckling—the one that looks different from others—is more likely to be a melanoma, even if it doesn't exhibit the classic ABCDE or I features.

Individuals at risk for melanoma should be examined by a physician on a regular basis. Regular self-exams are prudent as well. Examine your body in front of a mirror and use a hand mirror to view your neck, scalp, back, and buttocks. Report any suspicious findings to your dermatologist.

COMMON SKIN INFECTIONS

Fungal and Yeast Infections

Fungi and yeast all too often view our skin as fertile pasture; when these organisms decide to take root, their presence is made known in a variety of ways, some decidedly more unpleasant than others. Yeast inhabit skin and mucous membranes, and fungi colonize virtually everywhere, including the hair and nails. The many varied conditions caused by fungi and yeast follow.

Ringworm

More than a few grandparents can remember classmates in elementary school sent home because of ringworm. Few knew exactly what ringworm was, but it sounded horrible.

What is ringworm? Certainly not a worm! Ringworm is a contagious disorder of the skin or hair caused by a fungal infection.

Scalp ringworm is also called tinea capitis. As a rule, fungi will only infect the scalps of preadolescents. This is because at puberty the scalp oil glands begin to secrete substances that inhibit growth of virulent organisms. In other words, immunity to most fungal scalp infections is in place by the time one reaches junior high school.

Patchy areas of hair loss containing broken, fragmented hairs characterize tinea capitis. In more severe cases, these areas may contain scales and even pus-filled pimples. Ringworm is spread from person to person or may be caught from household pets, especially puppies and kittens.

Ringworm of the scalp is most commonly treated by the family physician, pediatrician, or dermatologist. Because the disorder is contagious to other children and may lead to permanent hair loss if left unchecked, treatment should commence as soon as the diagnosis is made. Scalp ringworm is treated with an oral medicine called griseofulvin, available in pill or liquid form. Therapy with this drug must continue for at least six weeks. In 2007 the FDA approved the drug Lamisil, in the form of granules that can be sprinkled on food, for the treatment of scalp ringworm.

Ringworm of the non-hairy skin, although more common in children, may also occur in adults. The causative fungi live on humans, animals, and soil. Body ringworm (tinea corporis) is characterized by red, scaly, circular patches that frequently itch. These patches characteristically have clear centers, hence the ringlike appearance. Tinea corporis may be spread by contact with pets and someone already infected. Nonprescription creams containing clotrimazole (Lotrimin), miconazole (Micatin), and terbinafine (Lamisil) are curative, although more extensive cases may require oral antifungal therapy as well.

Athlete's Foot

Athlete's foot (tinea pedis) is one of the most common fungal infections. Unlike body and scalp ringworm, this disorder is generally an ailment of adult life. You don't have to be an athlete to get athletes foot, but it sure helps. Fungi love sweaty feet, and they thrive on moist shower floors.

A fungal infection of the feet is characterized by itching, redness, and scaling. Severe cases may be accompanied by blisters. The condition most commonly occurs between the toes and may spread to the soles.

Prevention and treatment of athlete's foot entail minimizing excess heat and perspiration. Shoes and light socks that permit ventilation are recommended. Leather shoes and sandals are the best; plastic shoes and sneakers the worst. The feet should be thoroughly dried after bathing and then coated with a drying powder (talcum, Zeasorb, Desenex) before socks are put on. Mild to moderate cases can be controlled with antifungal creams; more severe cases may require oral antifungal agents.

Jock Itch

Ringworm of the groin (tinea cruris) is often found in men, especially in the summer months. The incidence in females is on the rise, with skintight slacks and panty hose being contributing factors. Conditions that predispose people to tinea cruris are moisture retention, heat, friction, and obesity. A red, itchy rash in the groin area characterizes jock itch.

Avoidance of tight, restrictive underclothing aids in the prevention and treatment of this annoying disorder. Drying powders that soak up excess moisture are also helpful. Cure may be obtained with antifungal creams, although reoccurrence is common.

Nail Infections

Fungal infections of the nails (onychomycosis) begin at the free margins and sides and result in yellowish discoloration, increased thickness, and brittleness. Toenails are more frequently involved than fingernails. The condition affects tens of millions of Americans, most between the ages of forty and sixty-five.

Because of the distortion and color changes, nail fungal infections are often a cosmetic embarrassment. Some may prove painful and interfere with walking. The condition is difficult to treat, requiring many weeks of oral antifungal therapy (Lamisil). Cure may be expected in about 60 percent of those treated. Topical therapy (Jublia, Kerydin and Penlac solutions) may prevent worsening but has an even lower cure rate. On occasion affected persons opt for surgical or chemical removal of an involved nail.

Tinea Versicolor

Ever look in the mirror and discover that your back and chest have become dotted with multiple scaling, discolored patches? No, the spots are not leprosy but are in all likelihood tinea versicolor.

Tinea versicolor ranks among the most trivial of all the disorders. This noncontagious condition is caused by a ubiquitous yeast-like organism that on occasion penetrates the outermost layer of skin, resulting in either light or dark flat areas characterized by fine scale. Tinea versicolor is most common in teenagers and young adults and is rare in children and senior citizens. Relatively few persons with tinea versicolor complain of itching; for the majority, the only complaint is a cosmetic one. Since the involved skin does not tan after sun exposure, the infection is most apparent in the summer months.

Tinea versicolor may be eradicated with a variety of different compounds including daily applications of selenium sulfide lotion (Excel, Selsun), ketoconazole shampoo (Nizoral) or a wide range of antifungal creams. Even with adequate treatment the discoloration may take months to normalize. Tinea versicolor infection is prone to reoccurrence.

Yeast Vaginitis

Yeast infection of the mucous membranes is called candidiasis or moniliasis. Yeast commonly reside within the vagina, but under certain circumstances, they may greatly increase in number, producing annoying symptoms. Vaginal yeast infections often occur during pregnancy and in diabetic persons. Certain antibiotics (especially tetracycline) and birth control pills may predispose to yeast overgrowth.

Candidiasis is characterized by a thin, white discharge accompanied by severe genital itching. Such symptoms should be investigated by a gynecologist, family practitioner, or dermatologist. Yeast vaginitis may be treated with antifungal creams applied in or about the vagina, vaginal tablets, and oral anti-yeast medications such as fluconazole (Diflucan). Women with recurrent yeast infections should be investigated for diabetes.

Paronychia

A paronychia is a swelling of the finger just below the nail. Many cases are associated with yeast infection. The tissue adjacent to the nail becomes red, swollen, and tender to the touch.

Paronychias are more common in women and frequently afflict persons who have their hands in and out of water, such as homemakers, bartenders, and hairdressers. No treatment will be 100 percent effective unless the affected site is kept absolutely dry. In other words, avoidance of moisture and irritants is usually necessary for complete cure. If wet work cannot be curtailed, gloves should be worn to protect the hands. Cuticles should not be unduly manipulated, and nail cosmetics are best avoided. Medical treatment consists of the application of antibacterial, anti-yeast, and anti-inflammatory creams or solutions three times daily.

Intertrigo

The inflammation that occurs wherever skin surfaces rub against each other is called intertrigo. The favored sites are the groin, under the arms and breasts, the buttocks, and between the toes. Contributing factors besides friction are heat, moisture, and sweat retention. Overweight persons are prone to develop intertrigo.

Intertrigo is characterized by redness, maceration, and irritation of the affected areas. In severe cases, the skin may weep and crack open.

Intertrigo is caused by a mixture of fungi, yeast, and bacteria. Treatment entails thorough cleansing and drying of the involved sites. The application of a topical anti-yeast cream should help resolve the condition. Use of medicated powders may prevent reoccurrence. Obese persons are urged to lose weight.

Bacterial Infections

Impetigo

An enormous number of bacteria reside on the skin's surface (would you believe four million microbes on just the hands!). Usually the germs peacefully coexist with the human host, but on occasion they invade beneath the skin and cause disease. Impetigo is a very contagious, rapidly progressing infection caused by either the Streptococcus or Staphylococcus bacterium. Preschool and school-age children are most commonly affected with this disorder, which has the highest prevalence in summer months.

Impetigo begins as a small, itchy, reddish area that rapidly develops pus-filled pimples that exude a sticky fluid. Within one to two days, a thick, adherent, golden-yellow crust forms over the entire region. The face is the most common location, especially around the chin and nose. If neglected, the infection may spread to other parts of the body.

Treatment of impetigo consists of applying warm water soaks to the affected sites three times daily, followed by the application of an antibacterial ointment such as mupirocin. This should be thoroughly rubbed into all patches. The patient and close contacts (other family members) should bathe daily with an antibacterial soap. Extensive, rapidly spreading cases require antibiotics taken by mouth and should always be evaluated and treated by a doctor. Adequate therapy quickly resolves the infection and prevents more serious consequences.

Cellulitis

Cellulitis is an acute bacterial infection characterized by a red, hot, well-defined, tender area of skin. The most common causative agents are streptococcal and staphylococcal germs, which may enter the skin secondary to minor trauma such as a scratch or insect bite. Growth and invasion of the bacteria produce inflammation, tenderness, warmth, and redness. The disorder is not contagious. Persons with diabetes are prone to developing this condition.

All cases of cellulitis should be evaluated by a physician. Hot compresses and oral antibiotics usually result in prompt resolution; if not, or if the condition is accompanied by elevated temperature, blood culture is recommended to rule out spread of the infection.

Flesh-Eating Bacteria: Necrotizing Fasciitis

Necrotizing fasciitis is an uncommon but serious bacterial infection that destroys skin along with fat and muscle beneath it. The damage is the result of toxins secreted by the bacteria.

Most persons who acquire the disease are in good health. The portal of entry may be as trivial as a small nick. Within twenty-four to thirty-six hours, the injured site worsens. Symptoms may include fever, chills, and excruciating pain. Immediate medical care and hospitalization are mandatory. Surgical debridement and IV antibiotics can be life-saving; indeed, some 30 percent to 40 percent of persons who contract necrotizing fasciitis die from the disease.

Boils

A boil is a localized skin infection caused by the Staphylococcus germ. The involved area develops a red, raised sore that is filled with pus. The sore is often sensitive to light touch. The skin thins out in the center, and a whitish-yellow point forms. This ruptures within two to four days, spilling out the enclosed pus.

Boils may form almost anywhere on the body but are most commonly encountered on sites of hair-bearing skin subject to friction and maceration such as the buttocks, neck, face, underarms, and thighs. Boils may be spread from person to person by close contact. Hence athletes participating in contact sports such as football and wrestling are prone to boils. Staphylococcal infections are readily passed to sex partners and to members of the same household.

Never squeeze a boil! Squeezing and picking at these sores may spread the infection and leave scars. Small boils are best treated with hot, moist compresses applied three to four times a day. The area should be frequently washed with a strong antibacterial soap such as Dial or Safeguard. When the boil begins to drain, pus should be removed as it forms and not allowed to contaminate surrounding skin.

An antibacterial ointment may be applied around the base of the lesion. Large boils, especially those occurring on the face, should be treated by the family doctor or dermatologist. He or she may wish to carefully open the boil, inject an anti-inflammatory suspension, and/or administer antibiotics internally by mouth. Towels, linens, and clothing used by a person with a boil should be kept separate until thoroughly washed.

MRSA

MRSA stands for *methicillin-resistant staphylococcus aureus*, and it is a growing problem in the United States. Although most cases occur in hospitals or other health care settings, an increasing percentage is being noted elsewhere, including high schools and colleges (often spread by contact sports such as wrestling and football). Clinically, lesions start as pimples that rapidly evolve into painful abscesses.

Suspected abscesses should be drained as soon as possible and cultured. Oral antibiotics may be required. The spread of MRSA is best halted by frequent hand washing or use of an alcohol-based sanitizer.

Lyme Disease

Lyme disease was first described in the mid 1970s. More than one hundred thousand cases have been reported, and it is the most commonly diagnosed insect-borne disease in the United States. The germ (classified as a spirochete) responsible for this disorder is transmitted to humans by the bite of a deer tick. The longer an infected tick remains attached to the body, the greater the risk of catching the disease. The first symptom of Lyme disease is usually an expanding red rash that resembles a bull's-eye. This appears one to four weeks after the tick bite and may measure several inches in diameter. The rash is painless and does not itch, but it may be accompanied by fever, chills, and joint pains. As the bacterium multiplies throughout the body, additional symptoms can include fatigue, severe headache, and even facial nerve paralysis (Bell's palsy). Advanced Lyme disease can result in neurologic deficits and persistent arthritis.

Lyme disease responds to oral antibiotics, and the sooner these are started, the better. Lyme disease should be considered a primary diagnosis for anyone with a history of a tick bite and the classic rash, as a specific blood test cannot be relied upon early in the disease. Preventative measures include wearing long sleeves and pants when walking through woods, use of insect repellants containing DEET, and the gentle removal of any tick (using a tweezers to pull the creature straight out) as soon as it is spotted.

Viral Infections

Herpes Simplex

Herpes simplex is a nasty virus capable of producing blisters on both the lips (cold sores) and the genitals. These sores are painful and unsightly and afflict millions of people each year. The virus is spread to others by intimate contact.

Cold Sore. A cold sore or fever blister is the result of a herpes virus invasion of the skin in and around the lips. The infection begins with pain or itching, followed by the typical fluid-filled blisters. The sores form a crust and dry up some seven to ten days later. Repeated attacks may occur because the virus burrows deep under the skin and "hibernates." Sunlight, emotional upset, and illness may awaken the virus and lead to new blisters. Some persons only develop a single episode; others are not so fortunate and develop recurrent blisters once a year or even as frequently as once a month.

Genital Herpes. Chances are great that a painful sore on the genitals is due to a herpes simplex infection. This is a venereal disease spread by sexual intercourse and oral sex. At the present time the condition is an epidemic, and the Centers for Disease Control estimates that over one million people become newly infected each year. It is believed that one in five American adults have been exposed to genital herpes.

Similar to the cold sore, a genital herpes infection begins with burning or itching, followed by blisters that crust over and finally disappear. The blisters may occur on either the male or female genitalia. Many cases, especially in females, occur without noticeable signs or symptoms, and some individuals remain unaware of their infection. Confirmation of infection is accomplished by a swab taken from an active lesion.

Genital herpes may lead to serious consequences in the newborn. A child born to a mother with herpes blisters at the time of delivery runs a high risk of catching the virus when exiting the birth canal. Such infection may prove fatal; thus, delivery by caesarean section is mandatory.

To date, herpes is incurable. Three oral medications (Famvir, Valtrex, and Zovirax) lessen the severity of each episode, and when taken on a daily basis, will lessen the frequency of attacks and the amount of viral shedding between outbreaks. Topical antiviral ointments (such as Denivir and Xerese) are much less efficacious. Various other treatment modalities, including lysine pills and dimethyl sulfoxide (DMSO), are without merit. All first episodes of herpes are best evaluated by a physician to ensure correct diagnosis and adequate counseling.

Herpetic lesions are best kept clean and dry. A topical anesthetic (for example, Anbesol Cold Sore Therapy) may temporarily relieve the discomfort. The annoying blisters of herpes dry up within a two-week period. Herpes is most contagious when visible lesions are present, and intimate, unprotected contact should be avoided during this period. Between outbreaks of genital herpes, condom use is prudent to prevent transmission.

People afflicted with herpes should derive some consolation in the natural course of the disease: as time progresses, the number of attacks subsides, and each episode diminishes in intensity and duration. Eventually the disease simply burns itself out. Those with herpes should remain hopeful that a cure will be found within the very near future.

For those who are sexually active and still herpes-free, caution and common sense are most certainly advised. Fear of herpes and the acquired immunodeficiency syndrome (AIDS) pervades our society and should play a major role in stemming promiscuity and unprotected sex. The majority of genital herpes infections are transmitted by individuals who are unaware that they are infected or show no signs of an outbreak. A vaccine is currently being tested on human volunteers, and its success could signal an end to the well-founded consternation over herpes.

Herpes Zoster (Shingles)

Herpes zoster, more commonly known as shingles, results in acute, painful blistering eruptions. The same virus that causes chickenpox produces this condition as well. Following a chickenpox infection, the virus hibernates in nerves under the skin, much like herpes simplex, to surface as herpes zoster in susceptible persons sometime in the future. Unlike herpes simplex, a person usually develops herpes zoster only once.

The onset of shingles is heralded by severe pain in a localized distribution. Because discomfort may precede the rash by some twenty-four hours, early diagnosis is sometimes difficult. (Indeed, herpes zoster of the chest is at times misdiagnosed as a heart attack!) Once the redness and blisters appear, the nature of the pain becomes quite apparent.

Complications of herpes zoster are infrequent but serious. Agonizing, persistent pain may remain about the affected area for weeks or months and is referred to as post herpetic neuralgia. Elderly persons are at greatest risk of developing this painful sequela. If the zoster virus invades the eye, blindness may ensue.

Most cases of herpes zoster should be evaluated by a physician. Herpes zoster infection usually does not signify an underlying abnormality, although persons afflicted with cancer and AIDS have an increased incidence. An ophthalmologist should be consulted if lesions approach the eye. Blisters may be treated with wet-to-dry saltwater compresses. Antiviral pills (Famvir, Valtrex, and Zovirax) will lessen the duration of an attack but unfortunately will not ward off post-herpetic neuralgia. Many cases warrant oral narcotic analgesia due to the severe pain.

Herpes zoster will occur in one out of every three individuals. Reactivation of the virus becomes increasingly likely with advancing age. A vaccine (Zostavax) stimulates antibody production and reduces occurrence of shingles by 50 percent and the risk of post-herpetic neuralgia by nearly 70 percent. The vaccine is recommended for most persons aged fifty and older.

Molluscum Contagiosum

Molluscum contagiosum is a viral disorder characterized by the appearance of pearly white to flesh-colored papules. Close inspection of each lesion usually reveals a slight depression (umbilication). The disorder is spread by skin-to-skin contact, and most commonly occurs in children, with lesions typically involving the face, trunk, and arms. In sexually active adults, molluscum are spread during sexual activity, and the lesions tend to localize to the upper thighs, lower abdomen, and genitals.

Molluscum will eventually disappear spontaneously, although persistence for over six months is not unusual. Because they are indeed contagious and often cosmetically unacceptable, treatment may be instituted early in their course. Molluscum can be physically removed in a doctor's office or treated with liquid nitrogen cryosurgery or the blistering agent Cantharone.

Viral Rash

Several viral diseases are characterized by fever and a typical body rash. The three most common are measles, German measles, and chickenpox.

Measles

Measles is a contagious disorder that begins much like the common cold, with nasal stuffiness and a dry cough. The skin eruption starts on the face and is accompanied by high fever. The rash spreads downward to involve the neck, trunk, and extremities and reaches its peak in three to five days. Most cases of measles occur in children, and this is indeed fortunate because the disease in adults can be quite severe. No specific treatment is available, but the disorder can now be prevented with a vaccine. Indeed, recent outbreaks in the United States highlight the importance of vaccination.

German Measles

The symptoms associated with German measles or rubella are usually very mild and include headache, fatigue, and slight temperature elevation. Shortly thereafter, a dusky red, blotchy rash appears on the face and rapidly extends to the trunk and extremities. Lymph nodes behind the ears are often enlarged and tender. German measles is not serious unless it occurs in a pregnant woman, in which case the results may prove disastrous. Rubella in pregnancy leads to eye defects, deafness, and heart malformations in the newborn. As with measles, German measles can be prevented with a vaccine.

Chickenpox

Chickenpox is another common infectious disease caused by a virus and characterized by a typical skin eruption. The disorder usually occurs in children and, as with measles, can be very severe in adults. Chickenpox begins with moderate fever and malaise, followed by an itchy skin eruption. The rash starts as pimples that rapidly become filled with fluid and surrounded by red at their bases (the configuration has been likened to "dewdrops on a rose petal"). Within four to five days, the lesions become crusted, although new ones may continue to form for about two weeks.

The number of cases of chickenpox has rapidly plummeted in the United States since the vaccine Varivax was introduced in 1995. Before the vaccine, four million Americans developed the disease each year, and over ten thousand required hospitalization. Children who haven't experienced chickenpox should get a first dose at twelve to fifteen months of age and a second between ages four and six.

Pityriasis Rosea

Pityriasis rosea is a common skin condition that affects people of all races and all ages, with the greatest incidence in adolescents and young adults.

The disorder begins with a single oval lesion covered with a fine scale. This is called the herald patch, and it is often mistaken for a ringworm infection. A few days later, smaller patches arise especially on the chest and back. On the back, the ovoid lesions follow the skin lines and are arranged in a "fir tree" distribution. Pityriasis rosea rarely affects the face. Itching, if present at all, is usually quite minimal.

The cause of pityriasis rosea is unknown. A virus is suspected, but the condition is not considered infectious (spread to others) or contagious (caught from others). Most cases seem to occur in spring and fall.

The mainstay of treatment is a simple reassurance. The condition is a nuisance but not serious. All lesions disappear entirely within three to eight weeks. Persons with extensive patches or bothered by itching may benefit from topical steroids and/or ultraviolet light treatments. Severe cases may warrant the use of oral steroids to hasten resolution. A recent study suggests that pregnant women who acquire pityriasis rosea during the early weeks of pregnancy have a higher rate of fetal loss.

HIV/AIDS

AIDS is an incurable disease caused by a virus and transmitted primarily by sexual relations and/or intravenous drug abuse. AIDS stands for acquired immunodeficiency syndrome; the virus (HIV) attacks the immune system, leading to marked debility and death. The disease is an epidemic with over one million cases reported in the United States. African Americans and Hispanics represent one-half of newly diagnosed cases.

The first signs of HIV frequently involve the skin. Infected persons may demonstrate white patches (thrush) within the oral cavity as a result of yeast overgrowth. Severe, persistent facial and scalp scaling (seborrheic dermatitis) may accompany HIV. Both psoriasis and herpes zoster (shingles) can also be triggered by the virus, and an HIV-positive individual is more prone to a multitude of ordinary and bizarre bacterial, viral, and fungal infections. One of the dreaded common features of AIDS is the appearance of violaceous patches and plaques of the skin surface called Kaposi's sarcoma, a form of skin cancer.

HIV infection is diagnosed by a blood test. In the mid-1990s, AIDS was a leading cause of death in this country, but newer therapies have dramatically decreased the death rate. Because there is currently no cure or effective vaccine, the key to curbing the spread of HIV is prevention. Practice safe sex and don't shoot up drugs.

Infestations

Scabies

Scabies is a contagious disorder characterized by itchy skin. The cause is a tiny mite barely visible to the eye as a minuscule speck. The creature is attracted to skin because of the warmth. The mite burrows within the top layer resulting in intense itching that is especially severe at night. Areas commonly affected include finger webs, wrists, buttocks, penis, and nipples. Red scratch marks and punctate bleeding points occur wherever the mite burrows. The face is rarely involved, except in infants.

Scabies is spread from person to person by direct contact. The condition readily infects other household members, sexual partners, and schoolchildren. Scabies has become epidemic in this country; over one million Americans each year contract the so-called itch mite.

Scabies is usually diagnosed by the characteristic physical appearance (multiple scratched pimples) and history of intense itching that is worst at night. Sometimes the burrows of the mite can be seen under a magnifying glass. A definitive diagnosis is made by microscopic examination of a skin scraping; visualizing the mite confirms scabetic infection.

Scabies can be eradicated using a prescription cream containing the ingredient permethrin. This should be applied over the entire body, except the face, for about eight hours and then thoroughly washed off. Lesions will clear in some two to three weeks. Treatment is advised for all persons in close contact with an infested individual. The oral medication Ivermectin will cure most cases of scabies as well.

Lice

Lice are bloodsucking insects that commonly infest the scalp, body, and genital areas. Their bite causes severe itching.

The scalp louse lays some three hundred eggs, each cemented to a hair shaft. Newborn lice must feed within twenty-four hours, or they will perish. Head lice usually affect children and are readily transferred among classmates; millions of school children are affected each year. Infestation triggers intense itching and scratching, which leads to open sores. Close examination reveals tiny white specks (nits) glued to the hair shaft.

Body lice may be transmitted by close contact or by wearing infested garments. The adult louse feeds on the skin, but lives within the seams of clothing. Most cases are associated with dirty, unsanitary living conditions.

Crab lice affect the hairy genital regions. They are spread by sexual contact and infest over one million Americans on a yearly basis. Thirty percent of infested persons will have another concurrent sexually transmitted disease. Crab lice result in ferocious itching of the genitals, which is especially severe at night. On close examination, the tiny louse may be seen as a brownish speck at the base of a pubic hair. Their eggs, or nits, are visible as small dots affixed to the hairs.

Lice are eliminated with medicated creams, lotions, or shampoos, although resistant cases have been reported. Resistance is an emerging problem with head lice. First-line therapy for head lice includes over-the-counter shampoos such as Rid or Nix and several prescription medications are available as well. Given that the nits hatch in several days, repeat treatment some ten days later is recommended with most therapies. Removal of nits is often impractical and not necessary but can be accomplished using special louse combs. Children with lice or their eggs do not need to be sent home from school.

Bedbugs

Bedbugs are on the rise, sparing no socioeconomic group. Several reasons for this are hypothesized including increased travel (hitchhiking in luggage), immigration, increased exchange of second-hand furniture, and resistance to common insecticides. Bedbug infestations have been documented in all 50 states. Although commonly associated with poverty and uncleanliness, the nasty critters occasionally make headline by setting up residence in some of the poshest hotels.

The bedbug bite goes unnoticed and intense itching develops later, the result of an allergic reaction. Often the bites are arranged in groups of three, appetizingly referred to as breakfast, lunch, and dinner. Sometimes the tiny buggers can be seen; wake up in the middle of the night and shine a flashlight on the bedsheets. The insects are small and flat, less than one-quarter of an inch in diameter. Infestation can also be recognized by the presence of red-brown specks (bedbug excrement) on sheets and mattress seams. The bugs can also live in cracks and crevices and under baseboards. Bedbugs avoid light and roam at night, drawn to a human host by body heat. They dine (suck blood) for five to ten minutes during which time their body weight swells some 200 percent, and their length increases by 50 percent.

A review published in the *Journal of the American Medical Association* notes that bedbugs fortunately do not transmit diseases. The problem is that, along with the severe itch, they do transmit fear and loathing.

Treating bedbug bites is easy. A topical steroid cream and oral antihistamines will do the trick. Ridding one's residence of these nasty critters is the hard part. Bedbugs can survive for up to a year after a single meal. Scrub infested areas with a stiff brush, and vacuum cracks and crevices. Use of special mattress bags will entomb the bugs and eventually kill them but will not rectify their using wall cracks and crevices as hiding places. Heat kills bed bugs and their eggs so entities such as clothes, bedding and stuffed animals are best placed in a clothes dryer set on the highest setting for at least 20 minutes. Bug bombs are not effective. A professional exterminator is often the best option and may require more than one visit.

PSORIASIS

Psoriasis is a very common disorder that affects up to 2 percent of the U.S. population. The condition may have a profound effect on the quality of life of those afflicted. In a study conducted by the National Psoriasis Foundation, over 60 percent of psoriasis patients expressed feelings of self-consciousness. As most cases begin before age thirty, individuals often require life-long therapy.

Psoriasis is characterized by red patches covered with a silvery, adherent scale. These patches usually do not itch. Any part of the body may become involved, but the most common sites are the elbows, knees, scalp, genitals, and lower back. Psoriasis may also affect the nails, producing tiny pits, discoloration, or marked thickening and distortion. Approximately 15 percent of psoriasis sufferers develop arthritis, which ranges in intensity from mild to crippling.

Psoriasis frequently begins in young adulthood, although childhood cases do occur. The course of the disorder is variable. In the summer months, the condition may improve, particularly following sun exposure. Worsening may follow a long illness or a period of stress.

The precise cause of psoriasis is as yet unknown, although abnormalities of the immune system play a seminal role. Heredity is also a factor, and people with close relatives who have psoriasis are more likely to develop the condition. Until recently, psoriasis was considered a disease of the skin and joints, and persons with the condition were believed to have the same general health as those without it. This concept has changed drastically during the past few years; recent studies have confirmed that persons with psoriasis are at increased risk of developing high blood pressure, diabetes, and myocardial infarction (heart attack). Whether this is due to the psoriasis, or to the fact that psoriatic patients have a higher rate of obesity, remains unanswered. Evidence is accumulating that the chronic inflammation associated with psoriasis has a deleterious effect on the heart and blood vessels.

Although no cure yet exists, psoriasis is a treatable disease, and good to excellent control is usually possible. Most cases respond to steroid ointments, creams, lotions, gels, sprays, or foams of which the most potent are betamethasone, clobetasol, and halobetasol. Tar is the oldest therapy and is derived primarily from coal. Drawbacks include odor and staining of both skin and clothes. Psoriasis of the scalp is commonly treated with tar shampoos (for example, DHS tar, Tarsum, and T/Gel) in combination with topical steroid lotions, gels, sprays, or foams. A vitamin A derivative, tazarotene (Tazorac), is FDA approved to treat psoriasis as are vitamin D derivatives (Dovonex, Vectical). Taclonex and Enstilar combine a topical steroid with vitamin D.

Natural and artificial ultraviolet light improve many cases of psoriasis. Combining ultraviolet A with the oral medication psoralen (PUVA therapy) may induce lengthy remission, but this therapy requires close physician monitoring and the use of a specialized light box. PUVA has been linked to the development of skin cancers. Emerging as a light-based alternative to PUVA is narrow-band UVB therapy. This also entails use of a light box, but no oral medication, and is believed to be safer in the long term. Treatments are ideally administered three times per week, and an average of thirty sessions is required to achieve maximum improvement. The excimer laser is approved by the FDA to treat psoriasis and emits a beam of light similar to narrow-band UVB. Multiple sessions are required, and insurance coverage may be an issue.

Individuals with extensive psoriasis who do not adequately respond to topical and/or light treatments may be placed on systemic therapy. The oral retinoid acitretin (Soriatane) is a potent derivative of vitamin A that can significantly reduce the severity of psoriatic plaques. Lesions usually improve within two months of commencing therapy. Since this medication can raise the level of circulating triglycerides (fats), periodic blood testing is recommended. Like isotretinoin the drug is teratogenic (may cause birth defects) and must be used with extreme caution in females of child-bearing age, and absolutely *never* by pregnant females

Methotrexate (MTX) is a potent oral medication used for more recalcitrant cases of psoriasis and for psoriatic arthritis. An advantage of MTX is that the entire dose can be taken once weekly. Favorable response is usually noted within six weeks. MTX can induce nausea, a low white blood cell count, and liver damage. Periodic blood testing is mandatory. A liver biopsy is sometimes recommended after prolonged use. MTX should not be used by pregnant females or those who cannot curtail use of alcohol.

Cyclosporine (Neoral, Sandimmune) is another oral medication commonly used for hard-to-control psoriasis. Response is often rapid, sometimes occurring within two weeks. The drug is taken daily and works by suppressing certain aspects of the immune system. Cyclosporine may raise blood pressure and serum lipid levels. It can also decrease kidney function, necessitating periodic laboratory monitoring.

A revolution in the treatment of psoriasis occurred in 2004 when the FDA approved Enbrel (Enteracept) to treat this condition. Enbrel is classified as a "biologic", a substance produced by human or animal protein rather than chemicals. All biologics are administered by injection and for many these are true miracle drugs markedly improving or even clearing skin, nail, and scalp disease. Many clinicians consider them safer and more efficacious than traditional systemic therapies with the greatest drawback being high cost.

Psoriasis is the result of a miscommunication between the immune system and skin. Signals are sent by specialized immune cells (T lymphocytes), inducing skin cells to multiply rapidly. The trigger mechanism for such behavior appears to be a combination of hereditary and environmental factors. Biologics work at the immune level, suppressing or altering the signals. Biologics are classified by their mechanism of action which will make little sense to the majority reading this book. To simplify: TNF alpha inhibitors include Enbrel (etanercept), Humira (adalimumab) and Remicade (infliximab). The first two are self-injected under the skin (analogous to insulin) and administered at home. The latter must be given by intravenous infusion (into the vein) at a medical center. Stelara (ustekinumab) is termed an IL12/IL23 inhibitor and it too is administered under the skin ("subcutaneously"). Stelara has an advantage of only requiring four injections each year. All are FDA approved to treat both psoriasis and psoriatic arthritis. In 2015 Cosentyx (secukinumab) became the first Il-17 inhibitor to reach the US market, followed in 2016 by Taltz (ixekizumab) and, in 2017, by Siliq (brodalumab).

In 2014 the novel agent Otezla (apremilast) was approved by the FDA to treat psoriasis and psoriatic arthritis. This drug is classified as a PDE4 inhibitor and is given by mouth twice daily.

Psoriasis affects millions of Americans. Recent medical advances ensure that virtually everyone with this condition can be significantly improved, and consultation with a dermatologist is highly recommended for those with this chronic disorder. Individuals with psoriasis are encouraged to contact the National Psoriasis Foundation (www.psoriasis.org) which provides a wealth of information on this subject.

ECZEMA/ATOPIC DERMATITIS

Atopic dermatitis, known to the majority of us as eczema, is a common skin disease that affects approximately one in two hundred people in the United States. In a recent survey, atopic dermatitis was found to rank among the ten most common skin conditions treated by the dermatologist. The incidence of this disorder is increasing, and it affects over 10 percent of children younger than fourteen years.

Eczema first appears in early childhood, often by the age of four months. The face, scalp, neck, and diaper areas are most frequently involved. These sites, especially the cheeks, become red and scaly. Itching is quite severe, and the infant may literally tear apart his or her skin, leading to bleeding sores and secondary infection. In most cases itching actually precedes the appearance of the rash; thus eczema is commonly referred to as "the itch that rashes."

As the child ages, the disorder tends to localize to the back of the neck, behind the elbows and knees, and on the wrists and ankles. The involved sites are dry and thickened, and demonstrate accentuation of the normal skin creases.

In the adult, atopic dermatitis may be manifested by scaling of the hands and feet, and by the appearance of circular, dry, scaling patches (called nummular eczema) anywhere on the body. Eczema at any age is characterized by moderate to severe itching.

Most persons with atopic dermatitis experience clearing of the disorder in their late twenties, and by age thirty a large number are free of disease. About 15 percent of persons with atopic dermatitis develop chronic localization to their hands (hand dermatitis).

The cause of atopic dermatitis is not fully understood. Hay fever and asthma are associated with this condition. Heredity certainly plays an important role as nearly 70 percent of atopic dermatitis patients have at least one other family member with eczema, hay fever, or asthma. Diet (food allergy) was thought to cause and/or aggravate the disorder, but this is unlikely except perhaps in the very early, infantile stage.

Atopic dermatitis is as yet without cure; the condition simply must burn itself out. However, the annoying manifestations can be controlled. Treatment of atopic dermatitis centers on control of the rash and, just as important, control of the itching. The more one scratches, the worse the disorder becomes and the longer it takes to heal.

People with atopic dermatitis should avoid any factors that aggravate sensitive skin. Fingernails, especially those of infants, must be trimmed as short as possible to avoid digging and tearing. Clothing should be soft, loose-fitting, and preferably made of cotton; wools and irritating synthetics are best not worn. Excess humidity and lack of it both promote itching and should be avoided. Over bathing and the use of harsh soaps contribute to skin dryness. One should use a mild, moisturizing soap and lubricating bath oil. Moisturizers should be applied to the skin on a regular and frequent basis.

Individuals with moderate to severe eczema warrant medical care by a dermatologist. Control of itching usually entails the use of steroid ointments and creams. Topical steroids are safe for long-term administration but should be used at a lowered potency if needed on a chronic basis. Oral antihistamines are commonly used, but of questionable value. Flare-ups may require oral or intramuscular steroids, and chronic, refractory cases in adults may need methotrexate or cyclosporine for adequate control.

Topical immunomodulators are often used to treat atopic dermatitis. Elidel cream (pimecrolimus) and Protopic ointment (tacrolimus) are non-steroid compounds approved to manage mild to moderate eczema. These may be used about the eyes and in the groin, problematic areas for steroids. To date, adverse effects from extended use of these agents have not been reported.

In 2016 the topical non-steroidal cream Eucrisa was approved to treat mild to moderate atopic dermatitis. This cream can be used on all body sites. The first injectable biologic to treat moderate to severe atopic dermatitis, Dupixent, was approved in 2017. Similar to all biologics, this medication is both expensive and revolutionary, a harbinger of other exciting therapies on the horizon.

In general, control of eczema begins with the use of more potent topical Steroids which are then tapered to less potent forms for maintenance, or to either Elidel, Protopic, or Eucrisa, all of which are steroid-free.

TOPICAL STEROID POTENCY EXAMPLES
HIGHEST POTENCY
Clobetasol propionate: Clobex/Olux/Temovate
Betamethasone dipropionate: Diprolene
Halobetasol propionate: Ultravate
Diflorasone diacetate: Apexicon/Psorcon
Fluocinonide 1 percent: Vanos

HIGH POTENCY
Triamcinolone acetonide: Aristocort/Kenalog
Desoximetasone: Topicort
Fluocinonide 0.05 percent: Lidex
Amcinonide: Cyclocort
Halcinonide: Halog
Flurandrenolide: Cordran

MEDIUM POTENCY
Hydrocortisone butyrate: Locoid
Hydrocortisonevalerate: Westcort
Mometasone furoate: Elocon
Fluticasone: Cutivate

LOW POTENCY
Desonide: Desowen/Desonate/Verdeso
Alclometasone: Aclovate

LEAST POTENT
Hydrocortisone 0.5% 2.5 %: Cortaid/Hytone

DISORDERS OF PIGMENT

Vitiligo

Vitiligo is a common skin disorder that affects about 1 to 2 percent of the population. The condition consists of one or more flat white spots on the skin that contain no pigment. The depigmentation may appear anywhere on the body in people of any age and any race. Most cases begin before the age of twenty years. The white spots are usually first noted on exposed areas of the skin or in the body folds, often during the summer months, following a suntan.

Vitiligo may remain stationary for years or may rapidly progress to involve a large portion of the skin surface. Areas of vitiligo produce no symptoms; however, because of the lack of pigment, painful sunburn readily develops with even brief sun exposure.

The cause of vitiligo is unknown, and the vast majority of affected persons are in good general health, although some cases are linked to thyroid abnormalities. The problem is basically a cosmetic one; the darker the original skin color, the more noticeable the condition is. The psychological effects are often devastating. Study has indicated that, in over one-half of all persons with vitiligo, the disorder has significantly impaired their ability to interact with others socially. Seeking advice from a mental health counselor or vitiligo support group is encouraged.

The treatment of vitiligo is not at all satisfactory, and the cosmetic disfigurement is often best managed by concealment cover-ups such as Covermark and Dermablend. These may be purchased in finer department stores, where aestheticians will match the coloring agent's shade with the individual's original skin color. Certain medications (called psoralens) in conjunction with sun or artificial light may enhance repigmentation but should only be administered by a dermatologist experienced with such therapies. Another light source, UVB Narrowband (Excimer laser), may afford comparable results and is easier to administer. Multiple treatment sessions are required. Early vitiligo may respond to topical treatment with potent topical steroids such as clobetasol or the calcineurin inhibitors Elidel and Protopic. A remedy for severe vitiligo is permanent depigmentation with the prescription topical bleaching agent monobenzone. This is a drastic step as the loss of pigment is irreversible and permanent. Michael Jackson was rumored to have undergone such therapy.

Individuals with vitiligo should always use a broad-spectrum sunscreen on affected areas; this will help protect the skin from becoming sunburned and from developing skin cancer.

Melasma

Melasma is a condition that presents as mottled brownish patches on the face. The most common sites are the cheeks, nasal bridge, forehead, and upper lip. The condition invariably affects women and is most common in more dark skinned ethnic groups such as Asians, Indians, and Hispanics. Melasma is believed to affect some six million women in the United States.

Several factors play a role in the development of melasma, including a hereditary predisposition. Hormonal changes are also implicated. Melasma occurring in pregnant females is referred to as chloasma (or "the mask of pregnancy"). Melasma may be induced or worsened by both birth control pills and exposure to sunlight.

Treatment of melasma, like vitiligo, is difficult. If the condition is related to pregnancy, gradual resolution may follow delivery. If the condition began while the woman was on birth control pills, discontinuation is often advised.

Protection from ultraviolet light is essential, and this should involve sun avoidance and sun protection utilizing daily application of a broad-spectrum sunscreen, the higher the SPF the better. This is important as window glass does not block out ultraviolet radiation of the A range.

Some cases of melasma will respond to a combination of sun protection and over-the-counter bleach creams, the latter usually containing low concentration of the agent hydroquinone (Esoterica, Porcelana). Higher concentrations (greater than 2 percent) are available by prescription. Hydroquinone inhibits an enzyme responsible for the production of melanin. Use of hydroquinone is somewhat controversial; in 2006 the FDA proposed banning this product from over-the-counter preparations in response to animal studies linking it to an increased risk of cancer.

Tri-Luma is a particularly effective topical agent. This prescription cream combines hydroquinone, a topical steroid, and tretinoin. Azelaic acid (Azelex, Finacea), tazarotene (Tazorac), adapalene (Differin), and glycolic acids also have skin-lightening properties. No matter what agent is chosen, response is slow, requiring a minimum of three months of therapy. Microdermabrasion may enhance the efficacy of topical agents. Lasers and chemical peels may prove of value but may also induce increased pigmentation.

Age Spots

Many individuals develop unsightly, perfectly flat dark spots on sun-exposed areas, especially the face and hands. Called "liver spots" by some, they have nothing to do with the liver. The spots are medically benign but cosmetically unsightly. Additional darkening may be prevented by sun avoidance and, when this is impractical, by use of broad-spectrum sunscreens. The lesions often respond quite adequately to liquid nitrogen cryosurgery and laser treatment. Besides the topical bleaching agents described above a number of skin "brightening" products are being marketed with ingredients such as niacinamide, bearberries, soy, licorice extract, vitamin C, kojic acid, and oligopeptide-34. Many are quite pricey—and of questionable efficacy—but appear safer than hydroquinone for long-term use.

HIVES

Surely all of us know at least one person (maybe even ourselves) who, after ingesting a certain food or medicine, has broken out in itchy bumps and patches. The condition is called urticaria, and it is a very common one, affecting over 15 percent of the population at some time during their lives.

Urticaria begins as a sensation of itching in a localized area. Minutes later the hive (or wheal) arises, lasting for minutes or hours before vanishing without a trace. Subsequent hives may appear anywhere else on the body, including the lips, mouth, genitals, and eyelids. Some hives may be induced by light pressure applied to the skin (dermatographism). Hives are caused by fluid leaking out of blood vessels located under the skin surface. Increased permeability of these vessels is the result of a chemical (histamine) released from specialized cells circulating in the blood stream.

Anaphylaxis is the most serious form of urticaria. Here the reaction is so widespread that even the throat and lungs are affected, swelling up and filling with fluid. Breathing may become impossible, and death from asphyxiation can result. Anaphylaxis is a life-threatening medical emergency.

Urticaria represents an allergic response and is most frequently caused by drugs, such as aspirin and penicillin; foods, with the most common being strawberries, shellfish, peanuts, and tomatoes; and insect bites, such as bee stings. At times the allergic agent (allergen) is difficult to track down; for instance, some cases of urticaria have been linked to food preservatives and dyes, others to hidden infection within the body (in these cases the body becomes allergic to certain germs or parasites). Some persons break out with hives when emotionally upset or when under stress.

If the cause of hives is not immediately known, one would do well to keep a detailed diary recording every single food item and drug that one ingests (including even over-the-counter preparations like aspirin). A record should also be made of each new wheal. Reviewing such a diary might enable one to pinpoint the allergen causing the hives.

People prone to or suffering from hives should avoid ingestion of citrus fruits, shellfish, and products containing aspirin, all of which can cause or worsen this condition. Such individuals should exercise caution when taking prescribed antibiotics, most notably penicillin and ampicillin, and would do well to notify a physician at the first sign of a rash.

The itching of hives may be relieved by cool-water or ice-water compresses. Oatmeal or cornstarch baths are quite soothing. Hives are treated medically with antihistamines. These compounds such as diphenhydramin (Benadryl) and hydroxyzine (Atarax) will often decrease or terminate the annoying symptoms. The major side effect from antihistamines is drowsiness, and one should drive and operate machinery with care. Often a better option is non-sedating agents such as Allegra, Claritin, or Zyrtec, all available without prescription. Some acute and/or persistent cases may also require oral or injectable steroid therapy. Persons experiencing wheezing or shortness of breath (anaphylaxis) must be rushed to the nearest doctor's office or hospital; a shot of epinephrine (adrenaline) may prove lifesaving.

In 2014 the drug omalizumab (Xolair) was approved for the treatment of chronic hives. Classified as a "biologic", Xolair is administered by needle under the skin once a month and tapered and/or discontinued when the condition improves or resolves. Results to date have been gratifying for many afflicted with this distressing condition.

IRRITANT AND CONTACT DERMATITIS

Inflammation of the skin that follows contact with an external agent may be produced in two different ways. In some instances, referred to as irritant dermatitis, the substance acts as a simple irritant causing direct damage to the skin. In the case of a contact allergy, a substance invokes an allergic reaction. Contact dermatitis results in nearly six million visits to physicians each year in the United States.

Irritant Dermatitis

Industrial workers, food handlers, dentists, bartenders, and homemakers frequently suffer from irritant dermatitis of the hands. Exposure of the skin to harsh soaps, detergents, solvents, and many other chemicals induces chapping and irritation with repeated use. Excess moisture promotes irritation by increasing the penetration of these substances. Initially the affected areas (most often the fingers, hands, wrists, and forearms) become red and itchy. Severe dryness, thickening, and cracking occur with long-standing exposure (a condition known colloquially as "dishpan hands").

Treatment of irritant dermatitis involves protection and rest of the involved area. Strict avoidance of excess heat, moisture, harsh soaps, and detergents is essential. Those affected should avoid unnecessary wetting of the hands. Because it is not unusual for irritant dermatitis to begin in the moist environment under rings that traps soap, chemicals, and dirt, all such jewelry should be removed before wet work. Specially formulated barrier-protectant emollients help to insulate the skin from environmental damage. Examples include Kerodex, Proteque, Tetrix and TheraSeal.

When washing the hands, use lukewarm water and, if possible, a mild cleanser such as Aquanil, Cerave, Cetaphil, or baby soap. Cleansers should be used sparingly and the hands thoroughly rinsed. Dry carefully with a clean towel, remembering to dry between the fingers. Plastic gloves or lined rubber gloves should be worn when washing dishes and clothes, when peeling or squeezing citrus fruits, and when in contact with harsh chemicals. Gloves should not be worn for more than twenty minutes at one time. If water happens to enter the glove, it must be removed immediately.

Affected hands should be lubricated with a skin cream or lotion several times during the day. Prescription preparations containing cortisone may be required in more severe cases.

Cosmetic Allergy

The average American adult is said to use at least seven different cosmetic products on a daily basis. An allergy to a cosmetic is manifested by redness, swelling, and itching wherever that substance comes into contact with the skin. If the offending cosmetic is a hair dye, irritated skin will develop around the ears and along the hairline. Should a woman become allergic to lipstick or lip gloss, dermatitis about the lips will ensue. An allergy to eye makeup results in swelling and scaling around the eyes, and an allergic response to perfume will occur at the sites where perfume has been applied.

In some cases, a person may use a skin care product for years without any problem and then suddenly become allergic to one of its ingredients. For this reason, one must always suspect an allergic reaction whenever inflammation of the skin develops in an area of topical application.

Should an allergic response be suspected, topical products are best discontinued. If the reaction subsides, it can be assumed that one of the eliminated products contains the offending agent. If necessary, to ascertain the offending product, possible culprits may be applied daily to the same small area of the arm, which should then be checked for signs of an allergic response. Alternatively, a dermatologist can test for an allergic reaction to specific ingredients by a simple process called patch testing, which consists of applying commonly found substances to the skin under an occlusive dressing kept in place for forty-eight hours, and then analyzed for redness and swelling. The most common ingredients that lead to allergic reactions in cosmetics are fragrance and preservatives.

The term hypoallergenic has been applied to a large number of cosmetics. Since nearly all cosmetics are carefully screened for allergic potential before marketing, most are indeed hypoallergenic and will not induce reactions in the majority of users.

Cosmetic Allergy: Common Culprits

Fragrances: Thousands of different fragrances are in use today in products such as perfumes, shampoos, soaps, deodorants, and moisturizers. Even products labeled "unscented" may contain masking fragrances. An allergic reaction typically occurs on the face and hands. When a spray such as a perfume is involved, redness and itching of the neck is classic as well.

Preservatives: Preservatives are used to extend the life of products and represent the second most common cause of contact dermatitis to cosmetics. Ingredients linked to preservative allergic reactions include quaternium-15, parabens, and thimerosal.

Hair dyes: Ingredient labels found on hair dyes request that users regularly test for allergic reaction prior to use. The most common allergen is phenylenediamine (PPD), the key ingredient in permanent hair dye. Allergic reactions may occur on the forehead and neck prior to affecting the scalp. PPD is also a commonly found ingredient in black henna temporary tattoos.

Nail products: Allergic reactions to nail polish and acrylic nails may present as redness and swelling about the nail. Touching the face and eyelids with the fingertips can induce a reaction at these sites as well. Causative chemicals include formaldehyde-based resins and acrylates.

Jewelry Allergy

Allergy to jewelry is quite common. A recent study has demonstrated that nearly one out of every ten females is sensitive to nickel. People with nickel allergy develop redness, scaling, and itching wherever this metal comes into contact with the body. Common sites include the earlobes (from earrings), upper chest and back (from bra straps), waistline (from belt buckles), and wrists (from watchbands or bracelets). Nickel allergy is on the increase in part due to the popularity of body piercings and the ubiquitous presence of this metal. In fact, nickel was designated "Allergen of the Year" in 2008 by the North American Contact Dermatitis Group.

Once a person becomes allergic to nickel, this sensitivity persists indefinitely. Thus, affected persons should avoid all prolonged contact with this metal. A chemical solution (dimethylglyoximine) may be applied to any piece of metal to assay for the presence of nickel. Many dermatology offices are equipped to test for this substance. Sterling silver, gold, and platinum earrings may be worn, but chances are great that costume and gold-plated jewelry contain nickel.

Nickel allergy frequently occurs following ear and body piercing. For this reason, body parts should be pierced with stainless steel instruments, and only stainless steel ornaments should be worn for at least the first month.

Plant Allergy

The most common plant allergy is due to poison ivy. Other offenders include poison oak, sumac, and the mango plant. All contain the same irritating chemicals, and all can produce itchy eruptions.

Plant dermatitis follows exposure of a body part to the leaves of an offending plant or to materials that have been in close contact with the plant, such as animal fur, tools, or clothing. Between twenty-four hours and one week following exposure, an itchy rash appears at the site of contact. Tiny fluid-filled blisters arise in patches and streaks. If the allergic material from the plant remains under the nails, poison ivy may be spread to unexposed areas by the fingers.

The best way to prevent any allergic dermatitis is through avoidance. Persons susceptible to poison plant allergy (this includes about 60 percent of the population) should be familiar with these plants and remain vigilant when gardening, camping, etc. When walking in wooded areas, wear pants, long-sleeved shirts, and socks. Poison ivy plants may be physically removed (wear gloves!) or chemically destroyed. Exposed skin should be thoroughly washed within fifteen minutes to avoid penetration of the noxious plant chemical. Specific barrier creams (such as IvyBlock) may afford adequate protection when applied prior to exposure.

Mild cases of allergic dermatitis may be treated with drying compounds such as calamine lotion and oatmeal baths. Severe cases of poison ivy, especially those affecting the eyelids, are best managed by a physician. Oral desensitization to prevent the allergic reaction of poison ivy is currently being tested but cannot be recommended at the present time.

Latex Allergy

Latex is a compound synthesized from the rubber tree. The use of gloves made with latex has increased tremendously over the past two decades given the concern over contracting such blood-borne diseases as hepatitis and AIDS. This increase in use has been paralleled by an increase in allergic reactions. The more one is exposed to latex, the greater the chance that an allergic reaction will develop. Thus this condition is encountered most frequently in health care workers, not unexpected, given that nearly 50 percent of hospital products contain latex.

The most common reactions to latex are either irritant or allergic dermatitis, generally localized to sites of exposure, mainly the hands. In some individuals, latex allergy has been linked to constriction of the airways (anaphylaxis) and to death from airway closure.

Although specific allergy tests are available, most cases of latex allergy are diagnosed by history. The cornerstone of management involves strict avoidance of latex. Use of latex-free gloves is mandatory for sensitive individuals, as is recognition and avoidance of other products that may contain latex, such as balloons and condoms.

DIABETES AND THE SKIN

The incidence of diabetes is increasing at an alarming rate in Western countries, this undoubtedly due to expanding bellies, sedentary lifestyles, and lack of exercise. The prevalence of this disorder has soared 30 percent in the past decade, and diabetes affects more than 6 percent of the US population. Approximately 25 percent of those twenty-four million Americans are undiagnosed. The abnormalities of blood sugar metabolism that characterize diabetes negatively impact not only the circulatory system and kidneys, but the skin as well. Skin manifestations related to diabetes affect many persons afflicted with this chronic disorder.

Individuals with poorly controlled blood sugar are prone to a variety of cutaneous infections including those caused by yeast (candidiasis) and bacteria (mainly staph infections). Most of these infections respond well to conventional therapies but tend to reoccur.

Of particular concern is any infection, abrasion, or ulceration of the lower extremities. Diabetics suffer not only from fragile veins and arteries (peripheral vascular disease) but also from nerve damage which results in loss of sensation in the legs and feet (peripheral neuropathy). Because of progressive nerve damage, a skin injury in a diabetic may not even be felt and can be readily overlooked, often with disastrous results. Even superficial foot injuries are prone to slow healing, infection, ulceration, and tragically, gangrene. Gangrene signifies the death of tissue, a prelude to amputation. People with diabetes have a 15 percent lifetime risk of developing lower extremity ulceration, and diabetics are well advised to have their legs, feet, and toes checked on a regular basis and to promptly seek medical attention for even the most trivial of injuries.

Diabetics commonly develop dark areas on the lower legs. This benign but unsightly condition is called diabetic dermopathy or shin spots. Such lesions are not painful and do not itch. They occur in over half of diabetics, most frequently in individuals over age fifty with long-standing disease. There is no effective treatment, and lesions may persist for years or spontaneously resolve. A smaller percentage of diabetics (less than 1 percent) are afflicted with necrobiosis lipoidica diabeticorum. This unsightly condition is characterized by the presence of waxy, yellowish-red patches and plaques generally localized to the lower legs. The condition is more common in women. Treatment is far from satisfactory, and the lesions, although asymptomatic, may ulcerate on occasion. Diabetics also may develop tense blisters of the feet (diabetic bullae), which are probably caused by increased skin fragility. The blisters usually heal uneventfully. Acanthosis nigricans is a skin condition arising on the neck and underarms. Affected areas develop a distinct black, velvety appearance. Individuals who are diabetic and obese are at greatest risk for acanthosis nigricans. The condition may dramatically improve following significant weight loss.

THYROID AND THE SKIN

The thyroid is a gland that resides within the lower neck and plays an important role in the regulation of many body functions through the secretion of hormones. Perhaps as many as fifty million Americans have some sort of thyroid disorder. The hair, skin, and nails are particularly susceptible to disorders of this gland. Interestingly, the gland also interacts with the immune system, and some individuals with chronic hives and vitiligo have antibodies directed against the thyroid.

When the thyroid is overactive, the gland produces too much hormone. Excess thyroid hormone leads to the condition called hyperthyroidism, which is characterized by sweating, fine shaking (tremor), weight loss, diarrhea, and heart palpitations. Affected individuals tend to feel hot and prefer cold surroundings. The skin becomes smooth, velvety, and moist. Itching can be generalized and persistent. Swelling and discoloration about the ankles, called pretibial myxedema, also occurs. Fingernails and toenails may become distorted and separate from the nail base. Treatment options include specific drugs, radioactive iodine, or surgery.

Too little hormone is indicative of the condition called hypothyroidism. Symptoms include fatigue, weight gain, cold intolerance, and constipation. The skin becomes cold, pale, dry, and coarse. Puffiness about the eyes is common. Nails become rigid and brittle, and hair markedly thins and may fall out in clumps. Wound healing is impaired; even a simple laceration may take longer than normal to heal. Treatment is accomplished using thyroid replacement medication.

Diseases of the thyroid require medical attention and are diagnosed by physical examination and an assay of circulating hormones in the blood stream. Both underactive and overactive thyroid disease can affect not only the skin but the heart and circulatory system as well. Some thyroid-induced skin changes may return to normal once adequate control is achieved.

AUTOIMMUNE DISEASES

On occasion, the human body becomes confused and starts rejecting normal tissue. This occurs as a result of antibodies directed against certain body parts. The antibodies are called autoantibodies (*auto* for "self"), and the resultant pathology is called autoimmune disease. Three types of autoimmune disorders, also referred to as collagen vascular disease, can have profound effects upon the skin.

Lupus

The autoantibodies associated with lupus may attack many organs including the kidneys, heart, joints, and central nervous system. Internal involvement represents the most serious form of the disease and is called systemic lupus erythematosus (SLE). Of note, 90 percent of individuals with SLE are females. The characteristic skin finding is the "butterfly rash," characterized by a well-demarcated zone of redness and dilated blood vessels situated on the nose and cheeks. This occurs in over half of SLE patients. The rash may be induced or worsened by exposure to sunlight or indoor tanning bulbs. Indeed, ultraviolet light can precipitate internal body organ flare as well. For this reason, all persons with SLE are urged to avoid UV exposure and, when this is not possible, wear a hat, long-sleeved shirt, and pants. Use of a broad-spectrum sunscreen is recommended as well.

A form of lupus that is confined to the skin is the discoid variety. Discoid lupus primarily involves the scalp, face, and ears and often begins as reddened, inflamed patches, which over time develop into discolored scars. When lesions occur on the scalp, permanent hair loss often results. Conversion of discoid lupus to the systemic form is rare.

As SLE may involve many organ systems, a coordinated multispecialty medical approach to management is often a prudent decision. Lesions of discoid lupus may respond to topical and intralesional steroids and are best managed by a dermatologist.

Scleroderma

Scleroderma is an uncommon skin condition characterized by hardening (fibrosis) of the skin and connective tissues. This is due to an abnormal production and accumulation of collagen. The most serious form, called systemic sclerosis, can involve internal organs such as the kidneys, heart, and lungs. Many patients experience an exaggerated response to cold, manifested as pain and color changes of the fingers. This is known as Raynaud's phenomenon. A localized form that affects only the skin is called morphea.

Systemic sclerosis, like lupus, frequently requires multispecialty management, which might include a rheumatologist, dermatologist, and internist. Morphea is best managed by a dermatologist.

Dermatomyositis

Dermatomyositis is a progressive autoimmune disorder highlighted by inflammation and degeneration of muscle tissue. This leads to aches and profound weakness. The characteristic skin finding is a reddish-purple rash (heliotrope rash) localized to the eyelids, cheeks, and nasal bridge. Papules may also arise on the knuckles (Gottron's sign). Most cases respond to high-dose oral steroid therapy. As with all collagen vascular diseases, affected individuals are urged to apply broad-spectrum sunscreens and wear protective clothing when outdoors.

SPORTS AND THE SKIN

Athletes are prone to a number of skin conditions, some trivial, others not so. As discussed, fungi, yeast and bacteria flourish in moist environments. Prolonged wearing of wet clothing following a workout will promote the growth of these microorganisms. Fungal spores shed from an individual with athlete's foot are readily transmissible from the floor of a damp locker room. Many cases of plantar warts (caused by a virus) are spread in similar fashion. Acne may be worsened by sporting activities that involve heat, pressure, and occlusion. Acne mechanica occurs under helmets and shoulder pads of football and hockey players.

Direct trauma can also affect the skin. Getting hit in the thigh with a line-drive baseball will of course result in a bruise. Constant rubbing of a sneaker against the foot may engender a friction blister. Friction from clothing and tight bras may result in irritation and even bleeding of the nipples ("jogger's nipples"). Tennis toe (subungual hematoma) is a painful traumatic condition that occurs when blood accumulates under the nail. Draining the trapped fluid will provide immediate relief.

Of course, outside temperature alone can directly affect the skin. A skier must be concerned about frostbite, a swimmer with acute sunburn. On cold, bitter winter days, layers of nonrestrictive clothing should be worn, paying attention to adequately protect the ears, nose, fingers, and toes. In the summer, sun protection for athletes should include a broad-spectrum sunscreen.

Swimmer's ear (otitis externa) is an infection of the outer ear canal. Children and teenagers who spend a lot of time in water are prone to this condition, as moisture promotes growth of the causative germs. Itching followed by pain are the main symptoms, and most cases will respond to topical antibacterial ear drops. Swimmer's itch is a completely different entity caused by a parasite that ordinarily affects birds and snails, but which can also burrow through the skin of humans. The parasite quickly dies but induces an allergic reaction in some people. Children are most often affected when swimming or wading in infested water. The disorder is quite benign, and the itchy rash will resolve spontaneously in a few days. Topical steroids will hasten resolution.

Fungal infection, in the form of a condition called tinea gladiatorum, can at times reach mini-epidemic proportions in high school and college wrestlers. The disorder is classic ringworm, with individual lesions characterized by redness and scaling. Banned from the mat with active lesions, wrestlers may take drastic measures to conceal them, including soaking with bleach and scrubbing with sandpaper.

Even more serious is herpes gladiatorum, a herpes simplex viral infection occurring in wrestlers. The blistering lesions cause pain and may be accompanied by fever, chills, fatigue, and swollen glands. Common to several infections in athletes, herpes is spread by skin-to-skin contact.

In December 2003 the Centers for Disease Control issued their first warning in regard to the growing number of competitive athletes diagnosed with the antibiotic-resistant staph infection MRSA. MRSA, which can resemble an ordinary boil, may be passed to other players through an open wound or skin-to-skin contact. Multiple cases have been documented in wrestlers and football players, but even fencers, cross-country runners, and field hockey players are at risk. Such infections have the potential to be serious health hazards. Contributory factors include physical contact, shared facilities and equipment, and poor hygiene. The CDC recommends covering all wounds, thoroughly cleaning all shared equipment on a regular basis, and washing hands at frequent intervals. Pass the ball, not the germs!

SKIN OF COLOR

Skin is skin, right? Well, not exactly. Some skin types are indeed more prone to various abnormalities. Skin of color constitutes a wide range of ethnicities and races including African-Americans, Hispanics, and Asians. By 2050, people of color will constitute half of this nation's total population.

Postinflammatory hyperpigmentation (PIH) is the name given to skin darkening that results secondary to trauma, such as a scratch, or from skin disorders such as acne and eczema. Acne is the most frequent skin condition in African-Americans, and the second most common problem in Asians. Some degree of pigmentation is normal, but in darker skin, color changes may persist and prove cosmetically unacceptable. The retinoids, including Differin, Retin-A and Tazorac, are helpful in preventing acne and will often induce significant lightening of darkened areas as well. Compounds containing the substance hydroquinone may also be effective. Lower concentrations found in products such as Ambi Fade Cream and Esoterica are available without prescription; concentrations above 2 percent usually require a doctor's prescription (brands include EpiQuin, Lustra and Nuquin). A sunscreen is generally advised for daytime use (sunlight may darken preexisting dark spots), and individuals are best advised that no matter which bleaching agent is used, significant lightening may takes months to become apparent.

Vitiligo is the result of pigment loss. Although this condition occurs in equal frequency among all racial and ethnic groups, the consequences are much more apparent in darker-skinned individuals. Treatment is difficult and may include prescription creams and ultraviolet light. Widely available camouflaging agents such as Covermark and Dermablend afford cosmetic relief.

Exaggerated scars called keloids may occur as a consequence of small abrasions, surgical wounds, or even ear piercings. Some keloids form from pimples, especially when situated on the chest, back, or neck (termed acne keloidalis). Keloids arise most commonly in black skin and may be cosmetically unattractive as well as painful. Injection of a steroid solution into the keloid can result in shrinkage. Surgical excision is also an option in certain instances, although the recurrence rate may be as high as 75 percent.

Razor bumps are also more common in African-Americans. Black hair is characterized by curved hair shafts. Following a close shave, newly emerging pointed hairs turn downward and pierce the surface of the skin resulting in irritation and bumps. This condition is called pseudofolliculitis barbae, and it affects approximately 50 percent of black men. Growing a beard results in cure; as the hair lengthens it lifts out of the skin. Use of a special straight razor or an electric razor may prevent recurrence. Electrolysis and laser hair removal are therapeutic options but require multiple treatment sessions.

SKIN FIRST AID

Burns

Burns may be caused by thermal, chemical, radioactive, or electrical agents. Burns are usually classified into the following three types:

A first-degree burn involves only the outermost layers of the epidermis and results in red, swollen skin that is tender and painful. This type of burn rapidly heals within one to two weeks without scarring. Examples of a first-degree burn include a moderate to severe sunburn or a burn resulting from a low-intensity heat source.

A second-degree burn extends below the epidermis to the dermis but does not involve deeper structures such as hair follicles. Second-degree burns are characterized by painful blisters and marked swelling. If left undisturbed, the skin heals within two to three weeks, again without scarring. Brief exposure to a hot liquid or curling iron might result in a second-degree burn.

A third-degree burn destroys both the epidermis and dermis. Because nerve endings are destroyed, severe pain is uncommon. Blistering, a function of dermal swelling, does not occur. Healing occurs slowly, often with marked scarring. Skin grafting is often required.

Minor, superficial burns may be managed without the intervention of a physician. Immediately following a burn, cold packs or ice should be applied to the burned area or the region may be immersed in cold tap water. Coldness relieves pain, reduces swelling, and limits the extent of damage. Best results occur if such therapy is instituted within one hour after injury. Trivial burns require no dressings or medications. If the skin is broken, application of a topical antibiotic is recommended.

The initial treatment of a chemical burn entails immediate, thorough irrigation with water. Depending on the chemicals involved, two to four hours of continuous washing may be required to limit the depth of injury. Neither chemical nor electrical burns are appropriate for self-care, and physician consultation should be sought as soon as possible.

Persons with burns of more than minor extent should be treated in a hospital emergency room where debridement and administration of a tetanus booster may be necessary.

Insects and the Skin

Most humans tolerate insects to a remarkable degree. However, when they start to feed on our skin and terrorize us with their stingers, tolerance rapidly dissolves. Several types of insects frequently abuse human flesh.

Bees

Bees pollinate flowers and manufacture honey. And occasionally, a nasty one will sting. Bee and wasp stings are painful and are rapidly followed by swelling and redness. Wasps and bumblebees ordinarily do not leave their stingers in the skin and can therefore sting repeatedly. The stinger of the honeybee, on the other hand, commonly breaks off in the skin, resulting in the insect's death.

If one is stung, it is best to flick the insect off the skin and not squeeze it. If the stinger still remains, it may be carefully removed with tweezers. Cold compresses or ice applied at the sting site may lessen the severity of the reaction. Calamine lotion or a medicated steroid cream may also afford some relief.

Less than 1 percent of persons are allergic to bee venom, but these individuals will encounter serious, life-threatening reactions if they are stung. Symptoms of generalized allergy include tongue and throat swelling, dizziness, and difficulty breathing. As 50 percent of deaths occur within thirty minutes of a sting, sensitive persons should carry an epinephrine injector (EpiPen) whenever outdoors in temperate weather. An allergist can administer desensitization injections to diminish the severity and danger of bee stings.

Mosquitoes

The ordinary mosquito bite produces an elevated bump that itches. A localized bite requires no treatment, although calamine lotion or cortisone cream may lessen the itching. In the tropics, mosquitoes transmit serious diseases such as yellow fever and malaria, but in this country they were generally thought to be mere nuisances until the recognition of the West Nile virus in 1999. Although infection is usually asymptomatic, about 20 percent of West Nile patients will develop flu-like symptoms shortly after being bit by an infected mosquito, and about 1 in 150 will experience severe neurologic disease, which may result in coma and lifelong disability. Mosquitoes also transmit Eastern equine encephalitis, which may be fatal.

In areas where mosquito disease spread has been identified, vigorous eradication endeavors are often initiated. Wearing hats and long sleeve clothing are of benefit. The gold standard of insect repellants is DEET used by millions of individuals for the past fifty years and certified as safe by the Environmental Protection Agency. The higher the concentration in a product, the better the protection. DEET is found in many products including Cutter, OFF!, and Repel. Some persons object to the odor and oily feel of DEET. Two other topical repellant compounds deemed effective against mosquitoes are oil of lemon eucalyptus found in Repel Lemon Eucalyptus and IR3535 (a synthetic version of a naturally occurring amino acid), found in Avon's Skin-So-Soft Bug Guard Plus IR3535 and Bullfrog's Mosquito Coast. BugBand Insect Repellent uses oil derived from geraniums imbedded in a wristband. The Don't Bite Me! Patch contains vitamin B1 (thiamine) which is absorbed through the skin and acts as a mosquito repellant. Insect Shield and Buzz Off are brands of clothing impregnated with permethrin, the chrysanthemum-based chemical noxious to many types of insects. Ultrasonic gadgets and bug zappers are ineffectual and a waste of money.

Spiders

Most spider bites cause minor swelling, redness, pain, or itching. Application of a corticosteroid cream may hasten resolution.

The two spiders that cause serious reactions in the United States are the black widow spider and the brown recluse spider. The black widow commonly nests in cellars, outhouses, and sheds. The dangerous female is recognized by a reddish-orange "hourglass" configuration on its belly. Within minutes following a bite, severe chills, vomiting, and cramps develop. Needless to say, such a reaction is a medical emergency and may necessitate hospitalization.

The brown recluse spider is widely distributed in the central and southern United States. It is a small, dark brown creature with a characteristic violin-shaped mark on its head. The spider hides in closets and drawers. A bite is followed several hours later by intense local pain and swelling. The affected area turns black, and gangrene may ensue. People bitten by this spider require prompt medical attention.

Ticks

Ticks suck human blood. Once on the body, a tick surreptitiously inserts its head under the skin and engages in its vampire-like activities. Undetected, a tick may remain at this site for days.

Ticks should be removed with care, firmly grasped with a tweezers and slowly withdrawn from the body. A tick should never be forcibly removed because the head will remain under the skin, producing a slow-healing sore. Following tick removal, the affected area should be washed with soap and then treated with an antibiotic ointment.

Ticks spread Rocky Mountain spotted fever, a serious disease with a high fatality rate. For this reason, anyone recently bitten by a tick who develops sudden fever, headache, or skin eruption should seek emergency medical consultation.

Ticks also spread Lyme disease, a condition characterized by a red, circular rash. One possible result of Lyme disease is arthritis, and for this reason, all suspected cases are best treated with antibiotic therapy.

Fleas

Fleas are an embarrassing problem, not so much to dogs and cats, but to people. These miniscule, wingless, bloodthirsty insects bite not only pets but humans as well; the bites cause red, intensely itchy bumps. Many pets, especially cats, are not sensitive to flea bites and, although infected, show no signs of infestation. The same goes for humans; about half of us are not sensitive (allergic), so an owner may not become aware of the problem until other family members begin to scratch.

Ridding one's pet of fleas is no easy task. Flea collars are the most popular but probably least effective means of pet treatment. Flea soaps and shampoos can kill adult fleas on animals but they do not provide lasting protection against reinfection. Potent dips and sprays, recommended by veterinarians, are the best treatment for your pet. Thorough cleaning and vacuuming, including carpets and pet bedding, along with pesticide aerosol bombs, are often required to treat an infested house. The itch of fleabites will be diminished by application of topical steroids. More extensive cases may warrant antihistamine therapy as well.

Chiggers

Chiggers are tiny reddish-hued mites that are difficult to see without a magnifying glass. Unlike ticks, they do not burrow but attach themselves to the skin and inject saliva containing digestive enzymes that break down skin cells. This process induces irritation and severe itching some twelve to twenty-four hours later. Raised reddened welts appear at the site, and these may last up to two weeks. Preferred areas are the ankles, armpits, belt line, and other skin folds. Chiggers fortunately do not transmit disease, but their bites can become secondarily infected.

Chiggers prefer warm weather and become inactive when the temperature falls below 60 degrees Fahrenheit. They live in grass and foliage. Wearing sleeveless shirts, shorts, and sandals or shoes without socks predisposes one to chigger bites in endemic areas. As they do not burrow under the skin, simply rubbing affected areas or bathing suffices to remove the critters. The itch can be alleviated by application of a topical steroid. DEET application will dissuade chiggers. The manufacturer of a compound called Chigg-Away claims that it both mitigates the itch and repels the bugs.

Dog, Cat, and Human Bites

At times, wildlife—certain people included—bite. Any bite that punctures the skin surface should receive medical attention. Each year over two million bites are reported, with dogs being responsible for some 85 percent of these cases. One-third of all animal bites occur in children, and about one-half of all bites are considered provoked. Bites account for about 1 percent of all emergency room visits. Approximately 1 percent of dog bites, and 6 percent of cat bites result in admission to a hospital.

Dog jaws are powerful and may induce crush injury, lacerations, and puncture wounds. Cat bites are usually of the puncture variety. Cat bites are three times more likely to become infected, as cats carry more dangerous germs in their saliva than dogs. All animal bites should be cleansed thoroughly with soap and water as soon as possible. Bleeding is best controlled by application of pressure. If the wound is swollen, apply ice wrapped in a towel. Obtain a history of rabies vaccination from the owner. If the owner is unknown, attempt to keep the animal in sight until animal control personnel arrive.

A cat bite, or more commonly a cat scratch, can induce cat scratch fever disease, which is caused by a bacteria. The condition begins as a reddened pimple at the site of injury, followed by the occurrence of painful, swollen glands and flu-like symptoms. Fortunately most cases are self-limited and resolve without treatment, although antibiotic therapy will shorten the duration.

Human bites too may prove quite serious, as the mouth is a reservoir for some nasty germs. Approximately 250,000 human bites are reported each year. Some occur as a result of fighting, others during playing. Regardless, any human bite that breaks the skin surface should be copiously cleansed with soap and water and monitored for signs of infection. Because of the potential for serious infection, many physicians will institute a three- to seven-day course of prophylactic antibiotic therapy.

CONCLUSION

Your skin. Bruised, bitten, and blistered. From bites to solar radiation, frigid blasts to searing heat, this resilient organ takes quite a beating. Molested by the environment, feasted on by teeming hordes of invisible microbes, and subtly traumatized on a daily basis, no wonder skin occasionally displays wear and tear.

In the search for longevity and lasting beauty, a good starting point is indeed your outermost cover. Be kind to your skin. It just may last a lifetime!

Printed in the United States
By Bookmasters